YOUR HOME DOCTOR™
Mom

Dr. Robert Fallis

Jennifer Boese
Shari Fallis
Caroline Matovic
Kevin Smith

THE MEDIUS PUBLISHING GROUP
USA • CANADA

Your Home Doctor™ - Mom
Copyright ® 1999 Dr. Robert Fallis

The publisher has used its best efforts to ensure that the contents of this book are accurate, and is sold without warranty of any kind as to the accuracy of the contents. The user accepts full responsibility for any consequence arising from the use of this book.

All women are unique, and this book is not intended as a substitute for the advice of your healthcare provider (whether this is your family doctor, gynecologist, obstetrician, midwife, pharmacist or a breastfeeding consultant, etc.) who should be consulted on all individual medical matters, especially if you show any signs of illness, unexpected changes, or problems.

The brand name products mentioned in this publication are trademarks of their respective companies. The mention of these products in this book in no way constitutes an endorsement of any kind for these products by the publisher of this book. The mention of these products in this book also does not constitute an endorsement by the companies that their products should be used in the way specified within this publication.

All rights reserved. No part of this book may be reproduced or transmitted in any form or by any means, electronic or mechanical, including recording, photocopying, or by any information storage and retrieval system, without the prior written permission of Dr. Robert Fallis and The Medius Publishing Group (Your Home Doctor Inc.).

All patient names used in this book are fictitious. Any similarity to actual individuals or events is purely coincidental.

Canadian Cataloguing in Publication Data

Fallis, Robert
    Mom

(Your Home Doctor™)
Includes bibliographical references and index
ISBN 1-894434-01-3

1. Postnatal care - Popular works. 2. Puerperium - Popular works.
3. Mothers - health and hygiene. I. Title. II. Series.

RG801.F34 1999   618.6   C99-931621-4

Book Design & Layout: Gordon Bate
Cover & Exercise Photography: Michelle Newberry

Printed in Canada

Published by The Medius Publishing Group,
a division of Your Home Doctor™ Inc.,
Suite 204 - 245 Pelham Road, St. Catharines, Ontario L2S 1X8
Web: http://www.yourhomedoctor.com

This book is dedicated to Mothers.

With the touch of your hand, the gleam in your eye, the smile on your lips, the warmth of your embrace, the size of your heart and the song in your voice, childhood becomes a magical time.

YOUR HOME DOCTOR
Mom

Acknowledgments

I sincerely thank all those who contributed, reviewed or otherwise provided support for this project. Your assistance, guidance and encouragement were invaluable. An extra-special thanks to Gordon Bate, who brought his artistic and organizational prowess as well as his integrity and a caring hand back to the project.

Chief Medical Editor/Author

Robert Fallis, BMSc, MD, CCFP

Contributing Authors

Jennifer Boese, RN
Shari Fallis, MD, CCFP
Caroline Matovic, RN, CLC
Kevin Smith, MD, FRCP

Contributing Reviewers

Kerry Boyd, MD, FRCP
Monique Bucko, RN, CLC
Carole Caron-Sheehan, RN, BEd, CPIC
Anthony Chan, MD, FRCS
Karen Freeman, SRN, SCM, RN, CPIC
Nancy Fung, MD, CCFP
Sheila M^{C}Donell, RN, CLC
Tracy Moorey, BA, CPT
Christina Plaskos, MD
Donna Rothwell, RN
Francine Walsh, RN, CPIC
Janet Warren, MD, CCFP

A special thank you to my loving wife, Cathy, who fed me, cared for me, entertained our kids and continually encouraged and guided me as I spent our weeknights, weekends and holidays in front of the computer.

Introduction

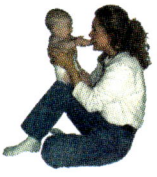

The development of **YOUR HOME DOCTOR**™ **for Mom** came as a natural extension of the *Your Home Doctor for Babies* book. What mothers wanted, we were told time and time again, was a book dealing with their concerns. Through daily encounters in our offices, clinics, call-in support services and focus group meetings, we discovered exactly what these common postpartum concerns were. We then set forth to deal with these issues in an experienced yet practical way.

This book is written by doctors, nurses, prenatal instructors and lactation consultants who are also parents. Many of the topics are written by mothers... for mothers. This provides an experienced "insider's" approach in helping you to understand what to expect and how best to deal with these problems.

You will find that anything that helps to make your life easier or saves you time as a new mom, especially in the first roller-coaster year, will be of benefit to you. That is the hope of this book. We were also advised that mothers needed a book that they could pick up and read quickly and easily when they happened to get a "break in the action". This includes bathroom breaks. Books with pages and pages of text, we were told, were intimidating and impractical for mothers. So YOUR HOME DOCTOR™ Mom was born!

In this book you will find that everything you need to know on a topic is generally found within two back-to-back pages. This is truly "meat and potatoes" medicine–that is, just what you are most likely to need to know.

This book also provides information in a variety of ways to try and accommodate the various ways that people learn and remember. These include the use of case studies, warnings, symptoms, goals and tips, and interactive flow charts. Knowing that people are often confused by medical jargon, we also include important definitions, synonyms as well as medications and treatments that may be of help with each condition. The "Trade Secrets" includes insider medical information or rules of thumb that let you know the "bottom line" when treating these medical conditions.

This book is not meant to be a textbook. It is rather meant to be a pre-textbook, or the first book you pick up when dealing with everyday postpartum concerns. The information it contains should help you deal with these problems in the comfort of your own home. This book will also advise you when you should abandon self-care treatment and head to the doctor, lactation consultant or the nearest emergency department.

Much of mothering is knowing about medical awareness and preparedness. This means being aware of any difficulties that you may encounter yourself or with your child. It also means being prepared for these common problems. I have found through my experience as an emergency and family physician that parents who are both aware and prepared seem to make the most outstanding parents.

I hope you find the information in this book provides you with a measure of reassurance in dealing with the many questions you will have as a parent. YOUR HOME DOCTOR™ Mom should also help clear up some of the unsound advice or horror stories people will have surely shared with you about motherhood and baby care.

The best advice anyone can give you is to develop and rely on your parents' intuition. Intuition is the innate sense or feeling that something may be wrong with your baby. This sixth sense develops shortly after your baby is born. Above all, learn to trust and believe in yourself. Mothers, I have found, are almost always right when they sense there is something wrong with themselves or their baby.

It is my sincere hope that this book will provide you with many practical solutions to common problems. May it become one of the many tools you can always rely on and trust during your journey into motherhood.

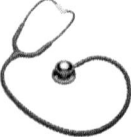

Dr. Robert Fallis

P.S.

I love to hear from mothers. If you can squeeze any spare moments out of your hectic schedule, your comments, questions and funny or heart-felt anecdotes are always welcome.

HEALTHY LIFESTYLE CHOICES

EXERCISE YOUR WAY BACK TO HEALTH

Helps reduce constipation, fatigue, back pain, urinary symptoms, urinary incontinence, depression and varicose veins. Helps improve strength and stamina, body self-image, sex, mood and sleep.

TAKE YOUR VITAMINS

Helps prevent and treat anemia and assures an adequate intake of essential vitamins and minerals.

USE A SEATBELT AND INFANT CAR SEAT

May be lifesaving to mother and baby.

REST FOR RECOVERY

Helps the body to cope with changes (physical and psychological) and increases your energy and endurance.

EAT A NUTRITIOUS DIET

Provides your body with essential nutrients to keep up with body demands and baby chasing. Follow the U.S. Food Pyramid or the Canada Food Guide. ***Remember, you need an extra 500 calories per day if breastfeeding.***

LEARN CPR AND FIRST AID

Increases awareness and preparedness for medical emergencies.

STOP SMOKING

Improves breathing and oxygen supply to mother and baby. Smoking is the leading cause of infant asthma and bronchitis and is a leading cause of death in women.

INCREASE YOUR FLUID INTAKE

Helps to prevent constipation, urinary tract infections and dizzy spells. Assists in your postpartum recovery.

GET PROFESSIONAL HELP

This doesn't mean just finding a doctor. You will also need to look into life, health, dental and disability insurance as well as wills and powers of attorney (both financial and medical).

How to Use This Book

This book is meant to provide practical advice for mothers dealing with common physical and emotional problems in their postpartum period. It is meant to do so in a clear, concise way to prevent busy mothers wasting their time flipping through pages of text to find the information they need.

By breaking down topics into bite sized pieces, including case studies, quotes, warnings, symptoms, goals, tips, flow charts, trade secrets, medication and treatments, definitions and synonyms, while sprinkling it with humor, we have attempted to provide you with all you need to know on each topic on four easy-to-read pages.

This book is by no means a text book on any of the subject areas, rather, it should be your first resource when dealing with these common postpartum concerns.

For those who can best identify with examples, I have written case studies for each of the medical conditions. They are written using the most common symptoms, signs, and scenarios to make them real for you.

Those who learn best with a conventional medical information style, will find the Warning, Symptoms, and Tip pages most helpful.

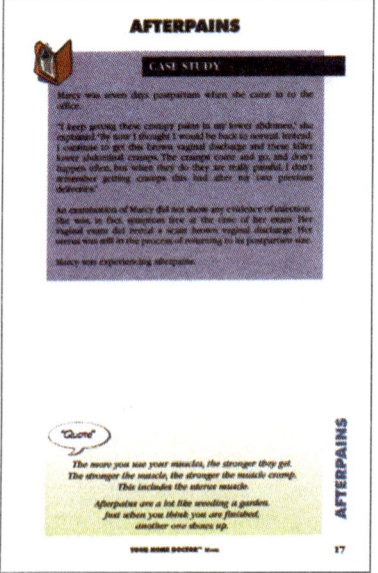

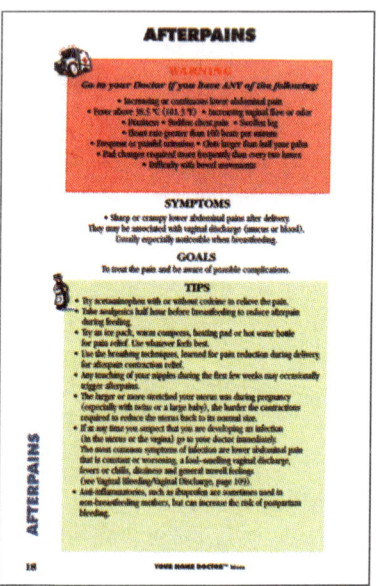

This book will help you to...

- Determine which conditions you are most likely to encounter.
- Define what it is about these conditions that you really need to know.
- Discover how to begin practical, safe treatment at home.
- Decide when to abandon home treatment and seek professional help.

Those who learn best with information in a visual format will find the flow charts the most helpful to diagnose and treat specific medical concerns.

Including "Trade Secrets", "Medications/Treatments", "Definitions" and "Synonyms", provides you with all that you require on treatment with a flip of the page. Synonyms are included because over the years I have found that people don't often understand the jargon used by the medical profession to explain diseases and treatments. Providing regular words to explain this jargon will help demystify the treatment process.

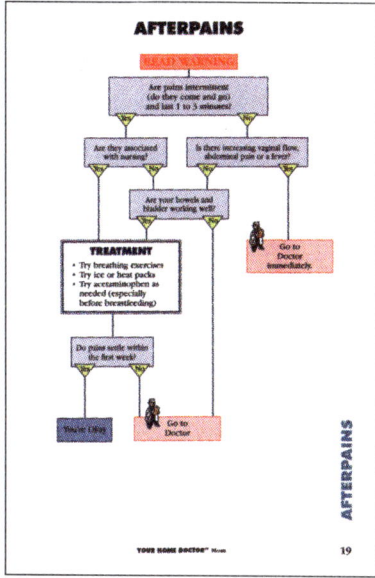

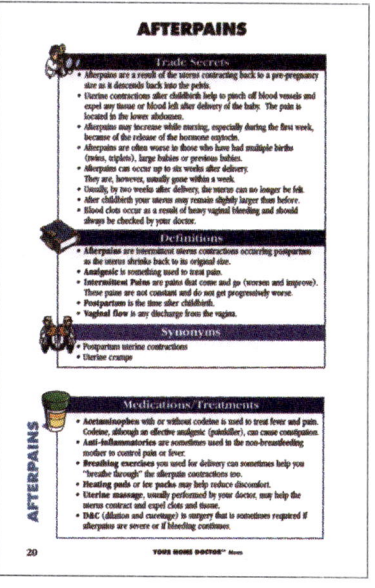

YOUR HOME DOCTOR™ Mom   13

CONTENTS

Foreword 5
Introduction 9
Healthy Lifestyle Choices 11
How to Use This Book 12

T O P I C S

- AFTERPAINS 17
- BACK PAIN & SCIATICA 21
- BIRTH CONTROL 25
- BODY IMAGE 29
- BREAST: ENGORGEMENT 33
- BREAST: INFECTION (MASTITIS) 37
- BREAST: PLUGGED DUCTS 41
- BREAST: SORE/CRACKED NIPPLES 45
- CESAREAN SECTION RECOVERY 49
- CONSTIPATION 53
- DEPRESSION 57
- EMOTIONS 61
- EPISIOTOMY AND PERINEAL CARE 65
- EXERCISE AFTER DELIVERY 69
- FATIGUE (TIREDNESS) 81
- HEMORRHOIDS 85
- MOTHERHOOD SURVIVAL STRATEGIES 89
- "NO-TIME" MANAGEMENT 93
- NUTRITION AND VITAMINS 97
- RELATIONSHIP CHANGES 103
- SEX CONCERNS 107
- SKIN PROBLEMS 113
- URINARY PROBLEMS 117
- VAGINAL BLEEDING AND DISCHARGE 121
- VARICOSE VEINS 125

CONTENTS

BREASTFEEDING
- Breast Feeding Benefits 129
- Positioning and Latching Your Baby   130
- Is Baby Getting Enough Milk? 133
- Feeding the Sleepy Baby 135
- The Breastfeeding Record 137
- The Breastfeeding Record Chart 138
- Pumping Breastmilk 139
- Storing Breastmilk 142
- Feeding Your Baby When You Are Away 143
- Weaning your Baby 145

BOTTLE FEEDING SUPPORT
- Bottle Feeding Benefits 147
- Bottle Feeding 149
  (Formula Feeding & Supplementing)

Your Postpartum Checkup (6 weeks) ...153

Coping: Your First Days at Home 154

Coping: Your First Weeks at Home 155

Birth Control 156

The Food Pyramid 161

Important Nutrients 162

The Bottom Line 164

Fatherhood Survival Strategies 165

The Home First-Aid Kit 169

The Home First-Medical Kit 169

Personal Information Chart 170

Record of Illness Chart 171

Important Numbers 176

AFTERPAINS

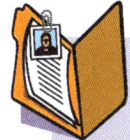

CASE STUDY

Marcy was seven days postpartum when she came in to the office.

"I keep getting these crampy pains in my lower abdomen," she explained. "By now I thought I would be back to normal. Instead, I continue to get this brown vaginal discharge and these killer lower abdominal cramps. The cramps come and go, and don't happen often, but when they do they are really painful. I don't remember getting cramps this bad after my two previous deliveries."

An examination of Marcy did not show any evidence of infection. She was, in fact, symptom free at the time of her exam. Her vaginal exam did reveal a scant brown vaginal discharge. Her uterus was still in the process of returning to its postpartum size.

Marcy was experiencing afterpains.

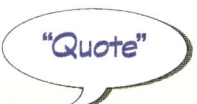

*The more you use your muscles, the stronger they get.
The stronger the muscle, the stronger the muscle cramp.
This includes the uterus muscle.*

*Afterpains are a lot like weeding a garden.
Just when you think you are finished,
another one shows up.*

YOUR HOME DOCTOR™ Mom

AFTERPAINS

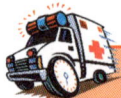

WARNING

Go to your Doctor if you have ANY of the following:

- Increasing or continuous lower abdominal pain
- Fever above 38.5 °C (101.3 °F) • Increasing vaginal flow or odor
- Dizziness • Sudden chest pain • Swollen leg
- Heart rate greater than 100 beats per minute
- Frequent or painful urination • Clots larger than half your palm
- Pad changes required more frequently than every two hours
- Difficulty with bowel movements

SYMPTOMS

- Sharp or crampy lower abdominal pains after delivery. They may be associated with vaginal discharge (mucus or blood). Usually especially noticeable when breastfeeding.

GOALS

To treat the pain and be aware of possible complications.

TIPS

- Try acetaminophen with or without codeine to relieve the pain.
- Take analgesics half hour before breastfeeding to reduce afterpain during feeding.
- Try an ice pack, warm compress, heating pad or hot water bottle for pain relief. Use whatever feels best.
- Use the breathing techniques, learned for pain reduction during delivery, for afterpain contraction relief.
- Any touching of your nipples during the first few weeks may occasionally trigger afterpains.
- The larger or more stretched your uterus was during pregnancy (especially with twins or a large baby), the harder the contractions required to reduce the uterus back to its normal size.
- If at any time you suspect that you are developing an infection (in the uterus or the vagina) go to your doctor immediately. The most common symptoms of infection are lower abdominal pain that is constant or worsening, a foul-smelling vaginal discharge, fevers or chills, dizziness and general unwell feelings (see Vaginal Bleeding/Vaginal Discharge, page 121).
- Anti-inflammatories, such as ibuprofen are sometimes used in non-breastfeeding mothers, but can increase the risk of postpartum bleeding.

AFTERPAINS

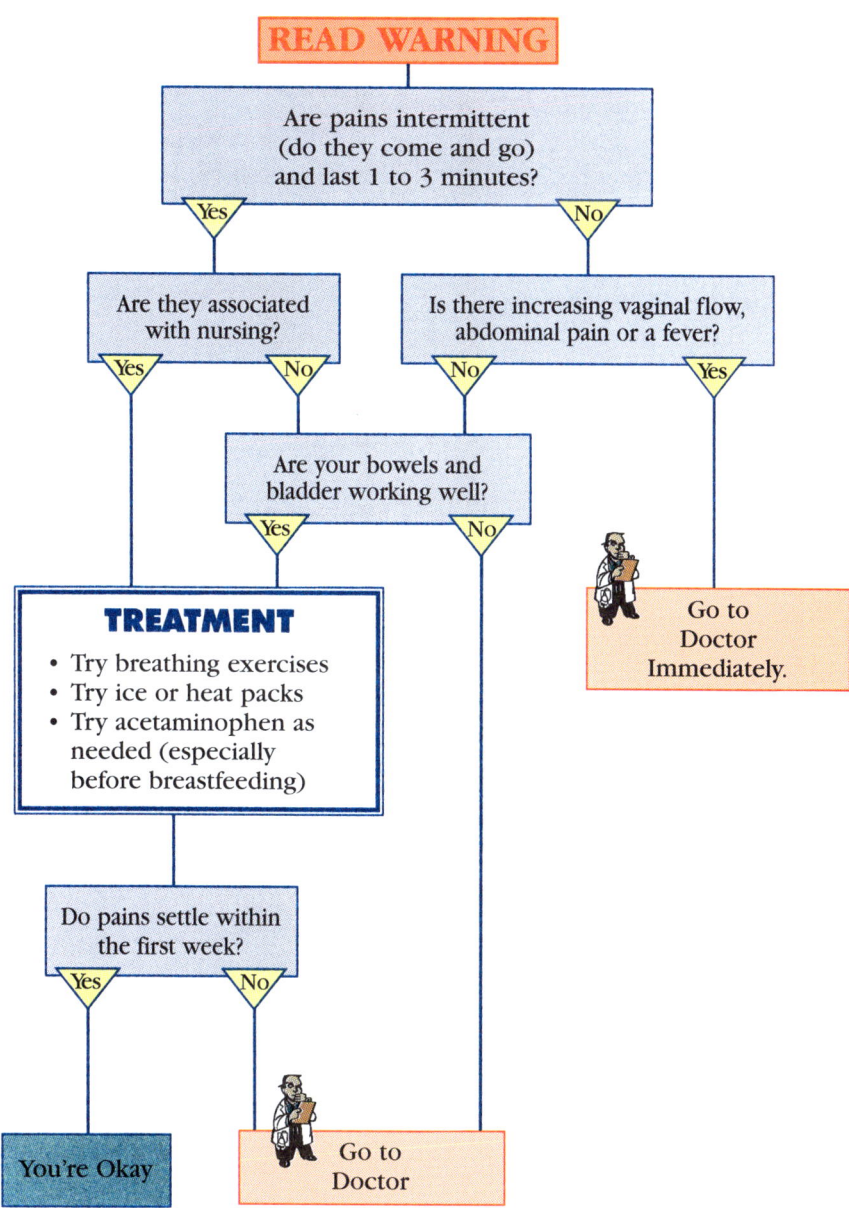

READ WARNING

Are pains intermittent (do they come and go) and last 1 to 3 minutes?

- **Yes** → Are they associated with nursing?
  - **Yes** → TREATMENT
  - **No** → Are your bowels and bladder working well?
    - **Yes** → TREATMENT
    - **No** → Go to Doctor
- **No** → Is there increasing vaginal flow, abdominal pain or a fever?
  - **No** → Are your bowels and bladder working well?
  - **Yes** → Go to Doctor Immediately.

TREATMENT
- Try breathing exercises
- Try ice or heat packs
- Try acetaminophen as needed (especially before breastfeeding)

Do pains settle within the first week?
- **Yes** → You're Okay
- **No** → Go to Doctor

YOUR HOME DOCTOR™ Mom

AFTERPAINS

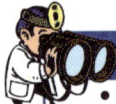

Trade Secrets

- Afterpains are a result of the uterus contracting back to a pre-pregnancy size as it descends back into the pelvis.
- Uterine contractions after childbirth help to pinch off blood vessels and expel any tissue or blood left after delivery of the baby. The pain is located in the lower abdomen.
- Afterpains may increase while nursing, especially during the first week, because of the release of the hormone oxytocin.
- Afterpains are often worse in those who have had multiple births (twins, triplets), large babies or previous babies.
- Afterpains can occur up to six weeks after delivery. They are, however, usually gone within a week.
- Usually, by two weeks after delivery, the uterus can no longer be felt.
- After childbirth your uterus may remain slightly larger than before.
- Blood clots occur as a result of heavy vaginal bleeding and should always be checked by your doctor.

Definitions

- **Afterpains** are intermittent uterus contractions occurring postpartum as the uterus shrinks back to its original size.
- **Analgesic** is something used to treat pain.
- **Intermittent Pains** are pains that come and go (worsen and improve). These pains are not constant and do not get progressively worse.
- **Postpartum** is the time after childbirth.
- **Vaginal flow** is any discharge from the vagina.

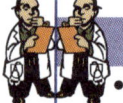

Synonyms

- Postpartum uterine contractions • Uterine cramps

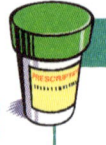

Medications/Treatments

- **Acetaminophen** with or without codeine is used to treat fever and pain. Codeine, although an effective analgesic (painkiller), can cause constipation.
- **Anti-inflammatories** are sometimes used in the non-breastfeeding mother to control pain or fever.
- **Breathing exercises** you used for delivery can sometimes help you "breathe through" the afterpain contractions too.
- **Heating pads** or **ice packs** may help reduce discomfort.
- **Uterine massage**, usually performed by your doctor, may help the uterus contract and expel clots and tissue.
- **D&C** (dilation and curettage) is surgery that is sometimes required if afterpains are severe or if bleeding continues.

BACK PAIN AND SCIATICA

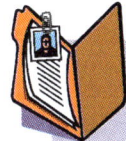

CASE STUDY

Marie-Anne was two weeks postpartum when she came in to the emergency department.

"I've had this aching low back pain ever since I delivered my baby," she explained. "Tonight when I bent over to put him in his bassinette I developed this sharp shooting pain down my left leg. I took Tylenol, rested on the couch and even tried applying ice packs to my back. My husband tried massaging my back and leg, but I just can't seem to get any relief."

Further history revealed that Marie-Anne had suffered low back discomfort in the past and her recent delivery had been fairly traumatic. She had experienced a failed use of vacuum suction and ended up requiring forceps to deliver a whopping 10 lb. 6 oz. baby boy.

Examination showed signs of nerve irritation without evidence of numbness, weakness or any bowel or bladder difficulties. There were obvious spasms in the low back muscles as well as some pain extending down the back of her leg to the foot.

Marie-Anne had developed back pain with sciatica.

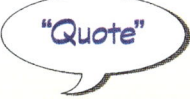

Back pain after having a baby is common.
Back pain after having quintuplets is assured.

Back pains usually resolve on their own,
with or without our help.

BACK PAIN AND SCIATICA

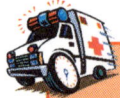

WARNING

Go to your Doctor if you have ANY of the following:

- Problems urinating or having a bowel movement
- Numbness, tingling or weakness of the legs
- Fever above 38.5°C or (101.3°F)
- Back pain that doesn't allow you to sleep, wakes you from sleep or is getting worse • Color changes, swelling or difficulty moving the legs
- Trouble breathing or chest pain • Abdominal pain

SYMPTOMS

- Discomfort of low back with or without pain, numbness or tingling extending down one or both legs.

GOALS

To determine the cause and relieve the pain.

TIPS

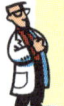

- Sleep on your side in a firm bed with a pillow between your knees, or on your back with pillows under your neck and knees.
- Apply heat or ice packs every hour for 15 to 20 minutes. Ice packs usually work best in the first 48 hours of back pain (helps stop the spasm and pain). Heat after 48 hours helps promote healing by relaxing muscular spasms and swelling.
- Try acetaminophen with or without codeine for pain.
- Try anti-inflammatory medications if not breastfeeding.
- Stand or lie down. Back pain is usually made worse by sitting.
- Wear supportive comfortable shoes with low heels such as running or walking shoes. Use an orthotic in your shoes.
- Sit in a straight-backed chair with a cushion in the small of your back. Try an orthopedic chair or an Obus forme back support. Try a hot bath or a massage.
- Avoid heavy lifting. Always lift by bending your legs not your back.
- Maintain good posture when sitting, standing, lying and walking.
- Use a maternity back support, girdle or Hara-obi to relieve pain.
- Try massage, physiotherapy or chiropractor treatment.
- Feeding baby may be difficult. Find a comfortable sitting or lying position with good pillow support. Wear a supportive nursing bra when not feeding.
- Swimming, yoga, tai chi and water exercises are excellent choices for reconditioning the back and body.
- Start exercises to stretch and strengthen the lower back once pain has started to settle. Do back exercises twice a day. Keep doing them even when your back is feeling better.
- Try TENS, acupuncture or ultrasound for pain control.

BACK PAIN AND SCIATICA

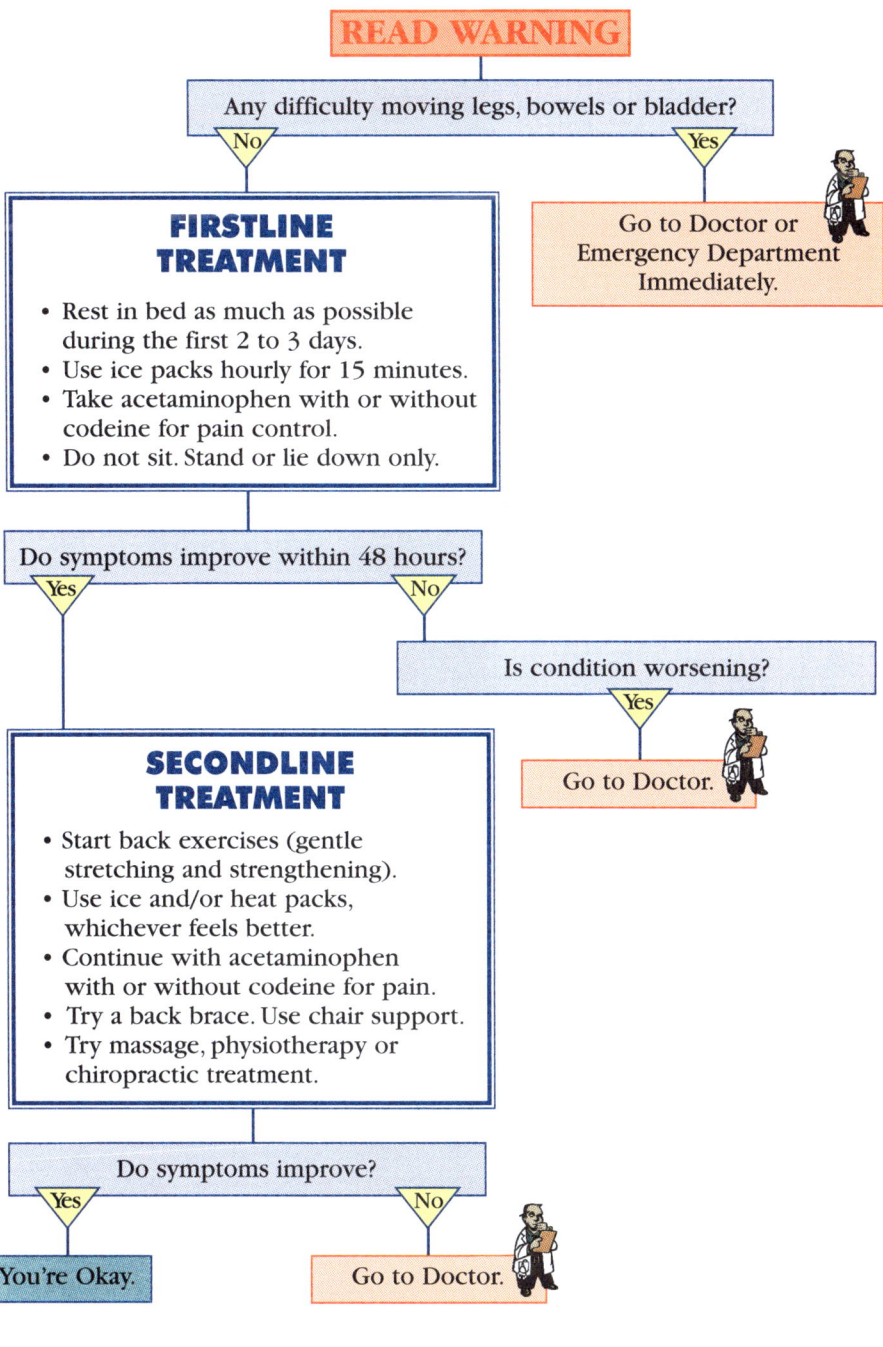

Beware of medications when breastfeeding.
Always check with your doctor before taking medicines.
This includes over-the-counter, herbal and naturopathic medications.

BACK PAIN AND SCIATICA

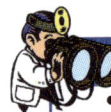

Trade Secrets

- Ligament relaxation from your pregnancy may make you feel weak, overly flexible and vulnerable to back injuries.
- Breastfeeding and carrying and lifting your baby often put additional strain on the back. Maintaining proper posture is extremely important.
- Stretch for spasms. Strengthen for aches.
- Avoid sleeping on your stomach or on a saggy bed. Lie on your back and place a pillow under your neck and knees to take the pressure off your back. Place a piece of plywood under a soft mattress to improve firmness.
- Exercises should always be low-impact.
- 80% of North Americans will be affected by back pain at sometime in their lives. 80% of back pains resolve on their own despite what we do.
- Only one percent of back pains end up requiring surgery.

Definitions

- **Low back pain** is commonly a result of muscle and ligament pain. Signs of nerve (neurologic) irritation include buttock or leg pain, numbness, tingling, weakness or problems urinating or having bowel movements.
- **Sciatica** are symptoms of the sciatic nerve irritation. Signs of sciatica include pain or numbness down the leg.
- **TENS** is transcutaneous electrical nerve stimulation.

Synonyms

- Back Spasm • Back sprain • Back strain • Low back pain
- Musculoligamentous low back pain • Nerve root impingement
- Sacroilialgia

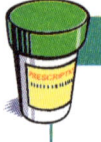

Medications/Treatments

- **Analgesics** such as acetaminophen with or without codeine are used for pain. Anti-inflammatories are also used for pain in non-breastfeeding women.
- **Exercise** helps to restore physical comfort by reducing muscle and ligament pain. Tai chi and yoga are excellent choices for treating low back problems.
- **Hot water bottles**, **heating pads**, or **heating packs** soothe muscular aches and pains.
- **Ice packs** ease acute back pain and spasm by helping to reduce swelling and inflammation.
- **Physiotherapy**, **chiropractic** and **massage therapy** can help when dealing with various back injuries.

BIRTH CONTROL

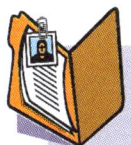

CASE STUDY

Mary Jane, 30, came to the office to discuss birth control options soon after the delivery of her second child.

Mary Jane and her husband, Bob, were still undecided about having a third child. They wanted to make their final decision in a few years, after their small business was successfully launched. Mary Jane had been on the birth control pill for ten years prior to her two pregnancies but now wanted to remain pill-free. Her periods normally lasted four to five days, with minimal cramping. She also wanted to breastfeed her baby for at least the first year.

Mary Jane decided to use an IUD for birth control. It was inserted at her 12-week postpartum visit to the office.

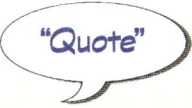

Parental fatigue following delivery is one of the world's most effective forms of birth control.
This form of birth control usually remains effective until the baby starts to sleep through the night.

Using breastfeeding as your only form of birth control may result in your early return to the delivery room.

Old joke: How can you tell which couple uses the rhythm method as their only form of birth control?...
They are the one expecting the baby.

BIRTH CONTROL

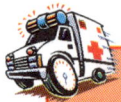

WARNING
Go to your Doctor if you have ANY of the following:
• Abdominal or chest pain • Trouble breathing • Leg pain or swelling
• Severe headaches • Numbness, tingling or weakness • Fever or chills
• Pregnancy • Unexpected vaginal bleeding
• Vaginal discharge or pain • Weight gain

GOALS
To understand the strengths and limitations of birth control methods., and to prevent an unwanted pregnancy.

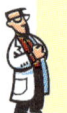

TIPS

- Talk to your doctor about the important features of the various birth control methods. This will help you decide what birth control option is best for you at this point in your life.
- Birth control methods can be designated as either permanent (if you never want to have more children) or temporary (if you want to control the timing of children in your family).
- Permanent birth control options are not considered reversible (e.g., vasectomies and tubal ligations).
- Temporary birth control options are reversible (e.g., condoms, foam, diaphragms, intrauterine devices, cervical caps, sponges).
- Temporary birth control options have varied effectiveness.
- Take your birth control pill approximately the same time each day. If you forget your birth control pill, take it as soon as you remember and use an additional form of protection.
- Only sterilization is 100 percent effective as birth control.
- Occasionally your body will expel the IUD. Check the string (found by feeling inside the vagina) regularly.
- Breastfeeding alone is not a good birth control option.
- There are now birth control pills that can be used during breastfeeding that are less likely to interfere with milk production.
- IUDs may be a good choice in women over 25 who have had a child and have only one sex partner.
- See doctor at six weeks postpartum for birth control advice.
- Women who have had an episiotomy or traumatic birth may need to try a variety of methods to find the one that is most comfortable for them.

BIRTH CONTROL

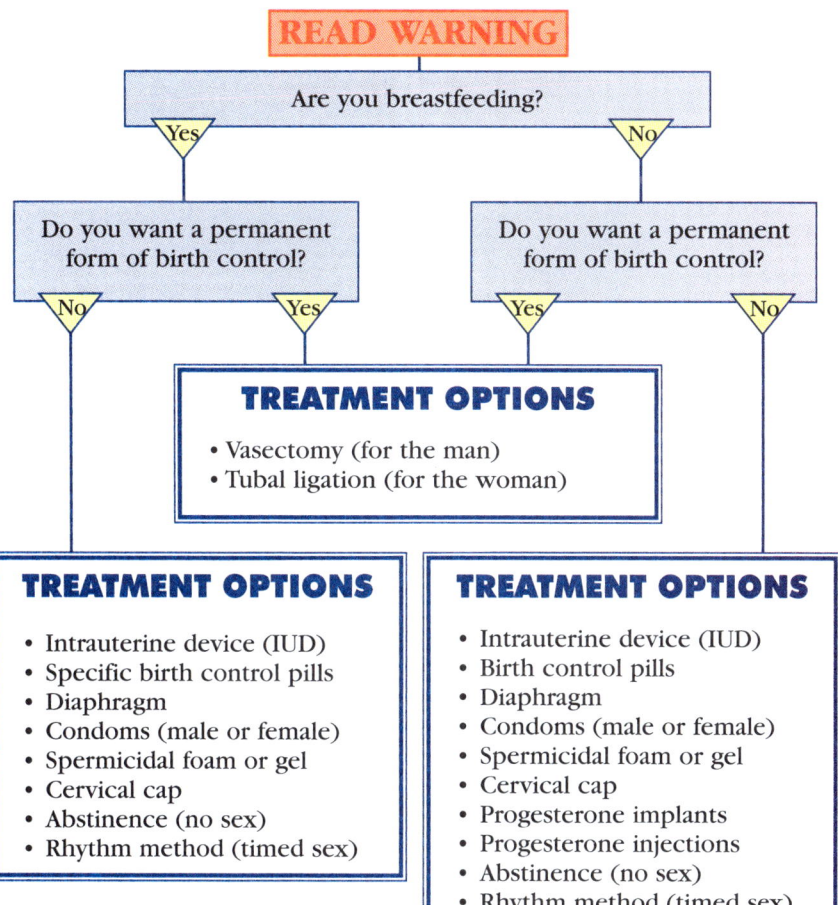

BIRTH CONTROL

Trade Secrets

- The best birth control method depends upon a person's medical history, life stage, beliefs, future plans and lifestyle.
- A woman may use several methods throughout her **reproductive years**. Talk with your doctor to help choose the best method for you.
- If you have any difficulties with your birth control pill, keep taking them but see your family doctor.
- YOU CAN GET PREGNANT WHEN BREASTFEEDING.
- Do not smoke if you take birth control pills.
- Always tell those treating you that you are on birth control pills. Certain medications will affect the birth control pill.

Definitions

- **Abstinence** is refraining from intercourse (sex).
- **Barrier method** is any form of birth control that intercepts (stops) the sperm from getting to the egg.
- **Progesterone** is a hormone used to control fertility. It comes in oral, injection and implant forms.

Synonyms

- Contraception • Family planning • Planned parenthood

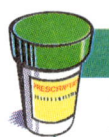

Medications/Treatments

- **Birth control pills** work by suppressing the release of the egg.
- **Condoms** (both male and female) prevent sperm from entering the vagina. They are also excellent for helping to prevent sexually transmitted diseases, including HIV.
- **Diaphragms/cervical caps** are round rubber domes that slip into the vagina before intercourse. These work by creating a barrier to sperm, preventing them from entering the uterus.
- **Hormonal implants**, six tiny progesterone-releasing seeds are inserted under the skin. They provide birth control for 5 years.
- **IUD** (intrauterine device) is a small plastic and metal device inserted into the uterus. It provides birth control for 2 to 5 years.
- **Rhythm** or natural family planning method uses timing, assessment of vaginal mucus and basal body temperature to help predict times of higher fertility.
- **Spermicide** is a sperm-killing cream, foam or gel that is placed in the vagina before intercourse.
- **Tubal ligation** is a hospital surgical procedure involving cutting or clamping the fallopian tubes that transport eggs.
- **Vasectomy** is an office surgical procedure involving cutting the vas, the tube that transports sperm.

BODY IMAGE

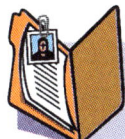

CASE STUDY

Wendy came in to the office three months after the birth of her baby.

"I knew it would take me a while to get back into shape after my baby, but it's been over three months and just look at me!" she gasped. "My belly still looks flabby and the stretch marks are disgusting. I'm worried I may never get rid of this extra fat! My goal was to get back into my old clothes before I go back to work next month. I want to diet but I'm still breastfeeding and I don't want the baby to suffer. To top it all off, someone in the supermarket last week asked me when the baby was due!"

Wendy's exam was medically normal. She had lost 20 of the 60 pounds that she had gained during pregnancy.

With reassurance and continued exercise, including stretching, strengthening and endurance work, she lost the remaining 40 pounds over the next nine months. Just in time for her next pregnancy.

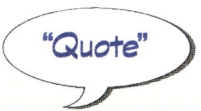

One of the most difficult things you will find as a mother is remembering to also take care for yourself.

What took nine months to create... may take nine months to correct.

BODY IMAGE

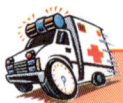

WARNING
Go to your Doctor if you have ANY of the following:

- A sense of losing control • Gaining rather than losing weight
- Low self-esteem • More bad days than good
- Symptoms of depression

(crying spells, decreased appetite, decreased mood and energy, poor sleep, feeling a lack of self-worth, poor concentration and memory)

- You are making yourself vomit or abusing laxatives

SYMPTOMS
- Feeling saggy, unhealthy, unfit, sluggish

GOALS
To reduce weight, tone muscles and regain pre-pregnancy form.

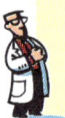

TIPS
- Breastfeeding will usually help you to lose weight faster. Check with your doctor before starting an exercise program. Exercise is usually not recommended until six weeks after delivery.
- Don't skip meals. Eat small and healthy snacks and meals every two hours throughout the day. This will help reduce cravings and prevent blood sugar levels from dropping.
- Try well-balanced reducing diets such as Weight Watchers.
- Increase fiber, fruit and vegetable foods and fluids.
- Consume six to eight glasses of water per day.
- Don't start smoking to lose weight.
- Don't use vomiting, laxatives or diet pills to help lose weight.
- Exercise daily while baby is napping. Try aerobic videos.
- To rid yourself of an abdominal paunch, you must tighten the abdominal muscles. Check with your doctor first.
- Use supportive bras to prevent breast sagging.
- Try tai chi or yoga classes for gentle stretching and strengthening.
- Try light weight training to improve muscle tone.
- Take a brisk walk daily with your baby.
- Socialize with others. Attend mom-and-tot exercise classes.
- Get out of the house daily with your baby.
- Get out of the house weekly with your partner.
- Take some time for yourself daily. This includes at some point every day enjoying a television program, a warm bath, reading a magazine, etc.
- Good grooming is essential in helping you feel good about yourself. This means daily showering, washing your hair, using make-up and putting on clothes. No days of pajamas, bathrobes and slippers allowed.

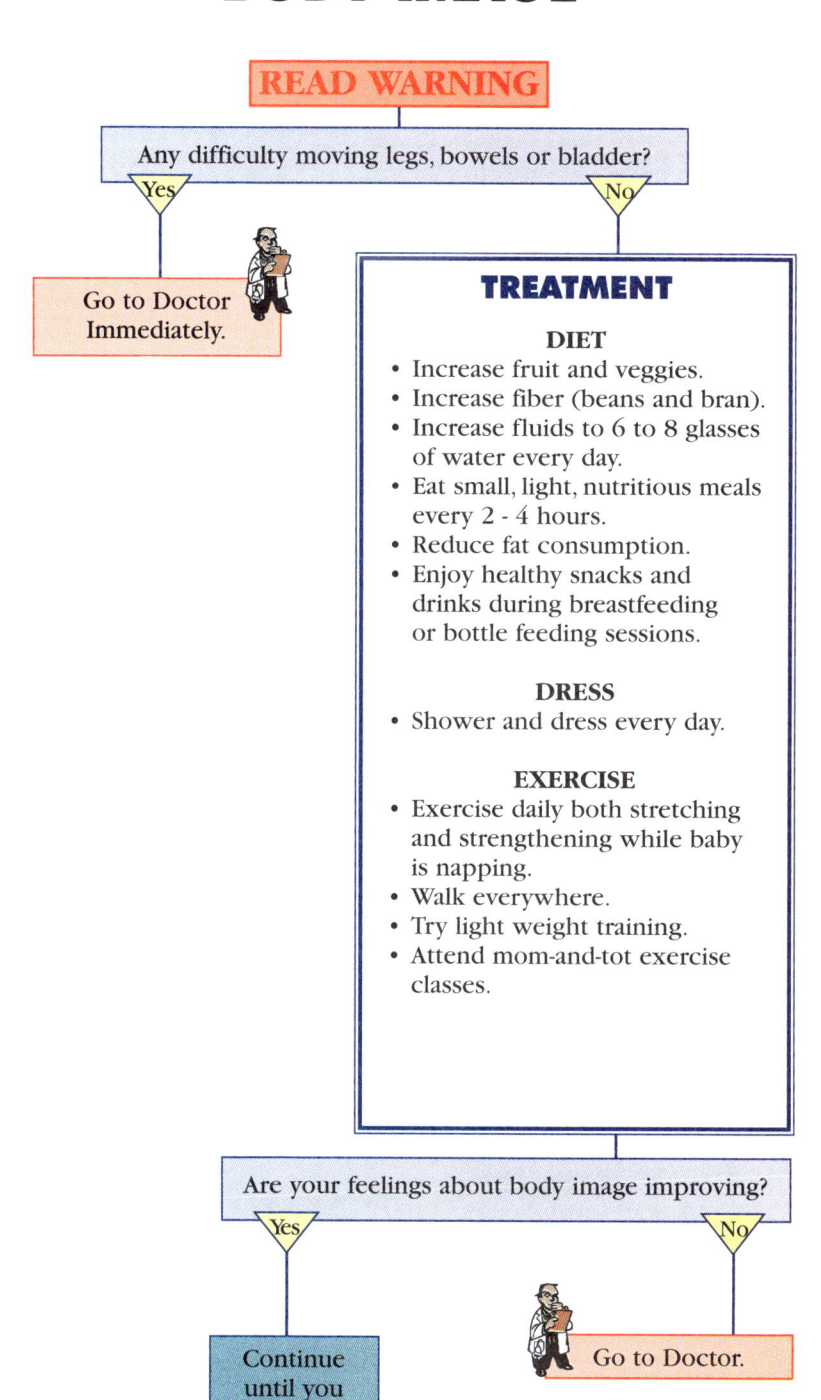

BODY IMAGE

READ WARNING

Any difficulty moving legs, bowels or bladder?

- Yes → Go to Doctor Immediately.
- No →

TREATMENT

DIET
- Increase fruit and veggies.
- Increase fiber (beans and bran).
- Increase fluids to 6 to 8 glasses of water every day.
- Eat small, light, nutritious meals every 2 - 4 hours.
- Reduce fat consumption.
- Enjoy healthy snacks and drinks during breastfeeding or bottle feeding sessions.

DRESS
- Shower and dress every day.

EXERCISE
- Exercise daily both stretching and strengthening while baby is napping.
- Walk everywhere.
- Try light weight training.
- Attend mom-and-tot exercise classes.

Are your feelings about body image improving?

- Yes → Continue until you return to normal.
- No → Go to Doctor.

BODY IMAGE

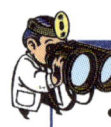

Trade Secrets

- The secret for good body image is good nutrition, good grooming and good exercise. Each is important alone, but together they help you feel great about yourself.
- Pregnancy and delivery is a life-altering event. You may not return to exactly how you were before.
- Breastfeeding helps reduce weight by burning up an extra 450 calories a day. This is equivalent to an hour of strenuous aerobic activity.
- It took nine months to accumulate fluids, fat and deconditioned muscle. It takes time to return back to normal. Some women remain an extra shoe or dress size larger forever after delivery.
- Socializing with other adults is crucial to your recovery.
- Get back to the pre-pregnancy or pre-delivery programs that you loved as soon as possible. Your outside interests are vital to your self worth.
- Motherhood is all about handling stress, compromising and being infinitely adaptable to the minute-by-minute changes. This includes learning how to cope with the changes in yourself physically, emotionally and spiritually.

Definitions

- **Body self-image** is your perception of how you look.
- **Depression** is an illness comprising a combination of both emotional and physical symptoms of hopelessness.
- **Fiber foods** are high in roughage (e.g., unmilled bran).
- **Self-esteem** is how you think about yourself.
- **Socializing** is enjoying companionship with others.

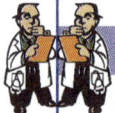

Synonyms

- Physical and emotional Self • Self-esteem

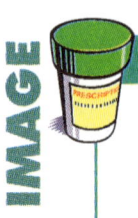

Medications/Treatments

- **Exercise** helps with toning, weight reduction and stress.
- **Psychotherapy** (counseling) is helpful for many psychological difficulties that may develop after delivery.
- **Weight-loss programs** (Weight Watchers, Jenny Craig, etc.) may help you get started with a healthy weight reduction.
- **Time management** is essential in helping you to balance new daily obligations and demands while still providing time for yourself (page 93).
- **Diet pills and laxatives** (medical and herbal) are ineffective and dangerous in weight reduction. Always check with your doctor before starting substances such as these.

BREAST: ENGORGEMENT

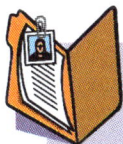

CASE STUDY

Julie was seen in the office four days after her delivery.

"I can't believe my breasts… they're so tender and hard," she groaned. "I don't think the baby is feeding as often as he should be, because my breasts are rock hard and he's having trouble latching on. Our feeding sessions have become screaming sessions for him and crying sessions for me. My baby has to eat. What can I do to get my breasts softened up for a little relief?"

Julie had been discharged as per hospital policy 24 hours after delivery. By the third day after delivery her breasts had begun to feel hard. Examination of Julie's breasts showed them to be swollen, hard and both warm and sore to the touch. The skin of her breasts had developed a shiny look. She did not have a fever, and no breast lumps were found.

Julie was suffering from a severe case of breast engorgement.

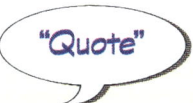

*Take a moment, ease the pressure,
pain relief will be your measure.*

*You will shed engorgement woes,
when your breast milk finally flows.*

BREAST: ENGORGEMENT

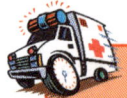

WARNING
Take baby to Doctor if you have ANY of the following:

- Severe breast pain • Chills
- Engorgement persists beyond 48 hours without relief
- Fever above 38.5°C (101.3°F) • Flu-like muscular aches
- Hot, red and tender breast, with or without a lump
- Red streaks on breasts
- You are concerned that your baby is not getting enough milk

SYMPTOMS
- Breasts feel painful, swollen and/or firm
- Breasts look red or "shiny" and may feel hot
- Nipples appear flattened or may be sore

GOALS
To relieve engorgement and maintain breastfeeding.

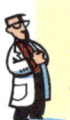

TIPS
For the Breastfeeding Mom
- Apply warm compresses to breasts or have a hot shower before each feeding. This will soften the areola.
- Feed baby frequently (every 2 or 3 hours) even during the night.
- Hand express or pump until the milk begins to flow or the areola softens enough for the baby to latch on.
- Breast massage during feedings may stimulate baby to feed longer, empty the breast better and receive more hindmilk. It will also help you find and "break up" any plugged milk ducts.
- If your baby does not nurse on an engorged breast during a feeding, hand express or pump to soften the breast enough to give relief.
- Apply cold compresses, ice packs or washed green cabbage leaves (with hard parts removed) to your breasts for 15 min. after each feeding.
- Avoid tight-fitting clothing, but wear a well-fitting, supportive bra (but not an underwire bra).
- Take acetaminophen, with or without codeine, for pain.
- Talk to a breastfeeding health professional early, for help.

For the Non-Breastfeeding Mom
- DO NOT pump or express milk from your breasts. This encourages your breasts to produce more milk and prevents your breasts from drying up. Engorgement goes when the breast milk goes.
- Apply cold compresses, ice packs or cabbage leaves as needed to relieve swelling.
- Wear a well-fitting, supportive bra. Avoid tight-fitting clothing.
- Take acetaminophen, with or without codeine, for pain.

BREAST: ENGORGEMENT

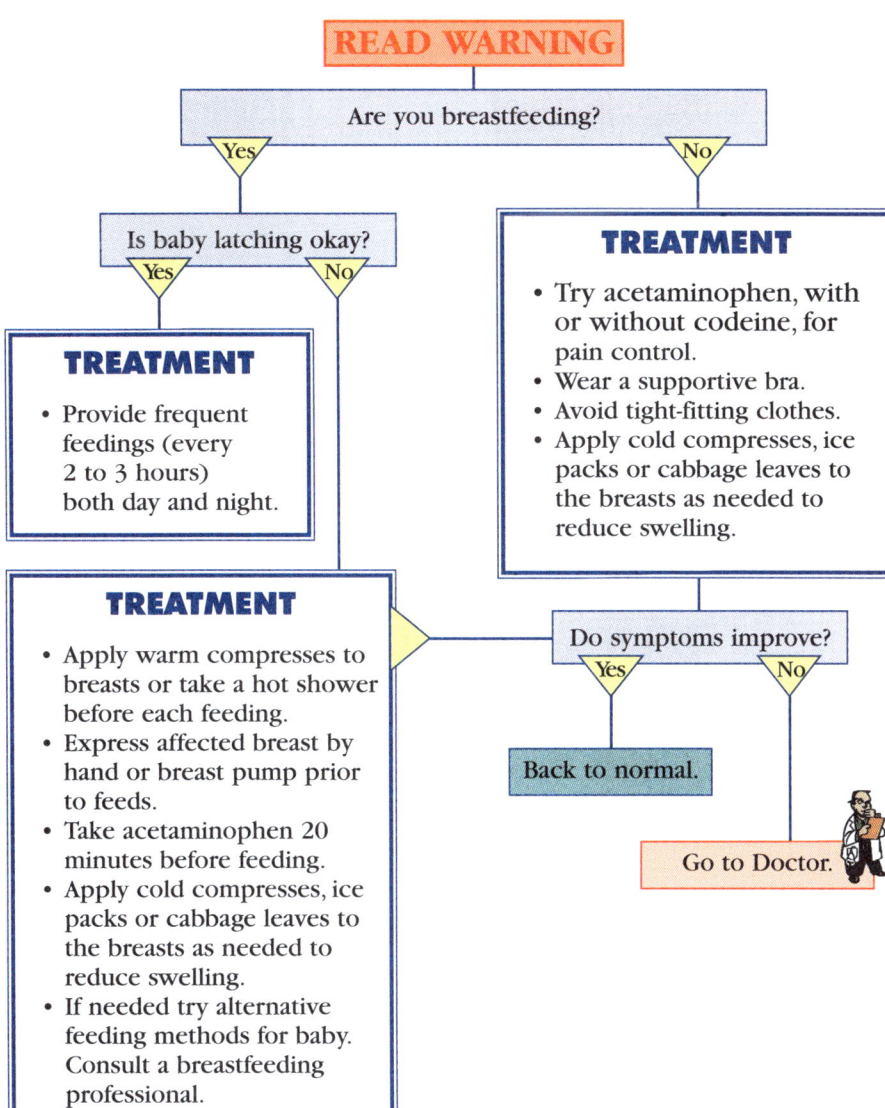

When to Get Help From a Breastfeeding Health Professional:
- *Engorgement is not relieved by suggestions from Tips section.*
- *Baby is not latching properly or you suspect baby is not getting enough milk.*
- *You have been told or decide to stop breastfeeding.*
- *Breast engorgement lasts more than 48 hours.*

BREAST: ENGORGEMENT

Trade Secrets

- Engorgement usually occurs when switching to formula feeding, weaning, when the latch is poor or when baby fails to adequately drain the breasts during each feeding.
- Engorgement is preventable and treatable through frequent feedings. Try to breastfeed every two to three hours (8 to 12 times per 24 hours) during the first few days after birth.
- Engorgement generally occurs on the third postpartum day and lasts for approximately 24 hours.
- See your lactation (breastfeeding) consultant early and regularly for breastfeeding problems. This includes any problems starting or maintaining breastfeeding or when considering switching to formula because of problems.
- Most doctors have not been taught the art of breastfeeding.

Definitions

- **Alternative feeding** is additional ways of feeding a baby. This includes supplementing with bottle or cup. Seek advice from your breastfeeding professional.
- **Areola** is the colored circular area around the nipple.
- **Breast engorgement** is distension and congestion of the breast.
- **Breast massage** is stroking of the breast to promote milk production and reduce plugging of ducts.
- **Hand expression** is milking the breast by hand.
- **Hindmilk** is the milk at the completion of a breastfeeding.
- **Latching-on** is the process by which the baby attaches to the nipple properly in order to breastfeed.
- **Let down** is the release of breast milk by the mother to baby.
- **Pumping** is milking of the breast by hand or machine.

Synonyms

- None

Medications/Treatments

- **Acetaminophen**, with or without codeine, is used to treat both pain and fever. Codeine improves pain control.
- **Anti-inflammatories/analgesics** (painkillers) are used for treating pain, fever or inflammation in non-breastfeeding moms.
- **Ice packs, cold compresses** or **cabbage leaves** are applied after or between feeds to reduce breast pain and inflammation.
- **Pumping/hand expression/showers** and **warm compresses** promote milk let downs, produce milk flow and provide pain relief.

BREAST: INFECTION (MASTITIS)

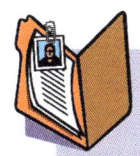

CASE STUDY

Karen was four weeks postpartum when she was seen in the office.

"I can't believe how lousy I feel," she stated. "My muscles ache all over, I feel hot, then chilled. If I didn't know any better I would swear that I'm coming down with the flu. I really haven't been sleeping well at all. Two nights ago was the first time that my baby slept through the night, but I was up four times. Could I be developing an infection somewhere?"

Examination revealed a sleep-deprived but otherwise positive and energetic woman. Her temperature was 38°C (100°F). She had a reddened area at the two-o'clock position on her left breast. It was just becoming tender to the touch. There was no lump although she admitted to having experienced plugged ducts twice since the baby was born. She had settled the problem previously by both feeding frequently and massaging the breast while the baby was feeding. Her armpit glands on the left side were also swollen and tender.

Karen had mastitis.

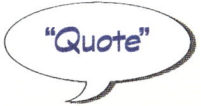

"Quote"

Cracked nipples are like an open invitation to an unwanted house guest – Mr. Bac Teria. Good old Anti Biotics will soon send him packing.

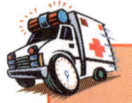

BREAST: INFECTION (MASTITIS)

WARNING
Go to your Doctor if you have ANY of the following:

- Increasing or severe fatigue • Flu-like muscular aching
- Fever (38.5°C or 101.3°F) or chills
- A localized hot, swollen, hardened, reddened and tender area on the breast
- Red streaks on the breast

SYMPTOMS
See Warning

GOALS
To prevent mastitis through early detection of plugged ducts. To identify and treat this condition quickly and to avoid breastfeeding complications.

TIPS

- Make sure the baby's latch is good (see Latching, page 130).
- Treat damaged nipples as soon as they occur (see Sore/Cracked nipples, page 45).
- See the section on Plugged Ducts (page 41).
- Rest and drink plenty of noncaffeinated fluids. The best fluids are water, juice and milk.
- Take acetaminophen for pain and fever control.
- Feed baby frequently on the affected side (this will hurt) to promote drainage. This will not harm or make your baby sick.
- Drain the breast through frequent feeding, massaging breast during feeding, pumping, or hand expression.
- Breastmilk may taste saltier when a mother has mastitis. If baby refuses to nurse off this breast, pump or hand express the breast to drain and maintain your milk supply. After a week on antibiotics, the normal flavor of breastmilk should return.
- Do not supplement breastmilk with formula, juice or water unless directed by your doctor. This increases the time between feedings. This may also increase your risk of developing mastitis or make mastitis worse.
- If your baby begins to sleep long stretches, consider pumping or hand expressing for comfort and to avoid mastitis.
- See your doctor early for antibiotic treatment!
- Take all of the antibiotics you are prescribed.

BREAST: INFECTION (MASTITIS)

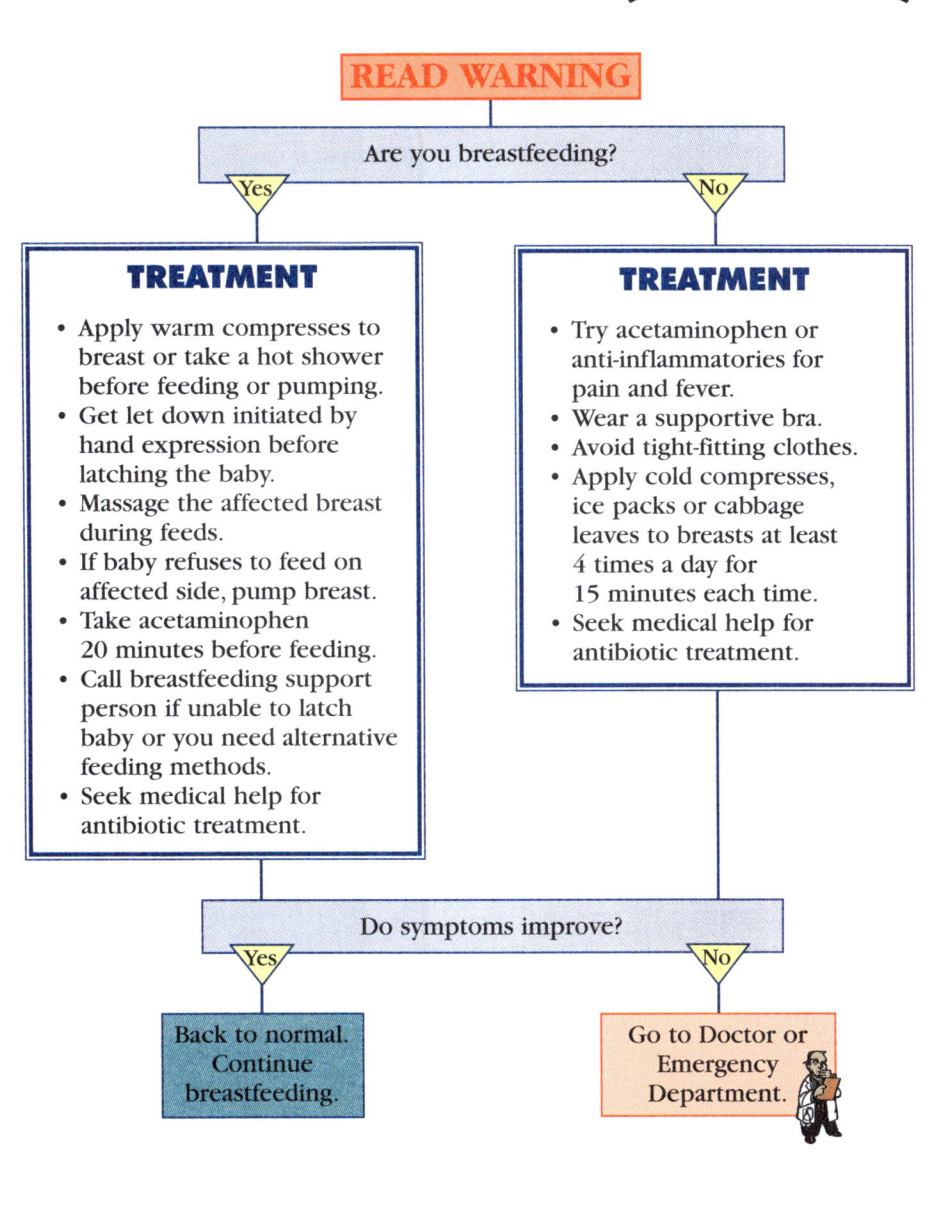

READ WARNING

Are you breastfeeding?

Yes → TREATMENT

- Apply warm compresses to breast or take a hot shower before feeding or pumping.
- Get let down initiated by hand expression before latching the baby.
- Massage the affected breast during feeds.
- If baby refuses to feed on affected side, pump breast.
- Take acetaminophen 20 minutes before feeding.
- Call breastfeeding support person if unable to latch baby or you need alternative feeding methods.
- Seek medical help for antibiotic treatment.

No → TREATMENT

- Try acetaminophen or anti-inflammatories for pain and fever.
- Wear a supportive bra.
- Avoid tight-fitting clothes.
- Apply cold compresses, ice packs or cabbage leaves to breasts at least 4 times a day for 15 minutes each time.
- Seek medical help for antibiotic treatment.

Do symptoms improve?

Yes: Back to normal. Continue breastfeeding.

No: Go to Doctor or Emergency Department.

BREAST: INFECTION (MASTITIS)

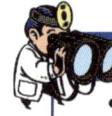

Trade Secrets

- Mastitis is usually preventable through proper latching, frequent feeding, meticulous care of damaged nipples, proper rest and the early detection of lumps in the breast.
- About 5% of breastfeeding women will develop mastitis.
- First-time breastfeeding moms are most at risk for mastitis.
- Breastfeeding during mastitis will not harm the baby!
- Mastitis should be treated with antibiotics.
- Mothers and babies are more prone to thrush when taking antibiotics.
- Other causes of breast or nipple pain include thrush infections and Raynaud's. Both require diagnosis and treatment by your doctor.

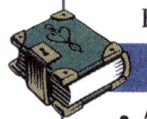

Definitions

- **Acidophilus**, or lactobacillus, is a bacteria found in yogurt or taken in capsule or powdered form. It acts as a friendly bacteria to reduce the occurrence of yeast infection (thrush).
- **Areola** is the colored circular area around the nipple.
- **Breast** abscess is a collection of pus in the breast that usually requires surgical drainage to cure the problem.
- **Mastitis** is an infection of the breast.
- **Raynaud's** is a blanching of the nipples from spasm of the blood vessels. It can cause sharp, burning or throbbing pain in the nipples. It may be caused by a poor latch.
- **Thrush** is a yeast infection affecting the nipples or breast. It can also be present in baby's mouth and diaper area.

Synonyms

- None

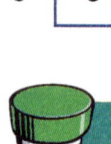

Medications/Treatments

- **Acetaminophen**, with or without codeine, is used to treat pain and fever. Codeine improves pain control.
- **Antibiotics** are used to treat infections. Only certain antibiotics are safe for the breastfeeding mother and infant. Always tell your doctor that you are breastfeeding.
- **Breast massage** during feeding helps to drain the breast and to clear plugged ducts.
- **Cabbage leaves** have been shown to be a safe, natural treatment for swollen, inflamed breasts.
- **Naturopathic products**, such as acidophilus, are sometimes used during a course of antibiotics to help prevent yeast infections. Consult a natural-food store for advice.

BREAST: PLUGGED DUCTS

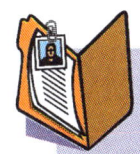

CASE STUDY

Sally came to the office at eight weeks postpartum.

"I was soaping my breasts in the shower yesterday when I found a lump on my right breast. I know that it is probably nothing or from my breastfeeding, but with the history of breast cancer in my family I thought it was important to have it checked out. Remember, my mother died of breast cancer at the age of 48".

Examination revealed a healthy but very concerned woman. Here breasts were normal except for a small lump at the one-o'clock position above the areola of the right breast.

Sally had a plugged duct.

The plugged duct, and lump, were relieved at the next feeding with breast massage.

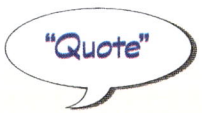

"Quote"

*Plugged ducts are a lot like traffic problems.
If you correct the blockage, you correct the flow.
If you correct the flow, you make everyone happy.*

*Preparation is thoughtful planning for the worst
while anticipating the best.*

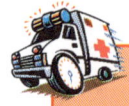

BREAST: PLUGGED DUCTS

WARNING
Go to Doctor if you have ANY of the following:

- A lump in your breast or a reddened area on your breast but you DO NOT have a fever, any flu-like muscular aches, chills or feelings of fatigue

SYMPTOMS

- Plugged duct may be red, tender or warm to the touch
- A lump may be felt if the plug is close to the skin

GOALS

To treat a plugged duct before it causes an infection.

TIPS

- Check your breasts daily for any lumps or any other symptoms of a plugged duct. It is often easiest to check while you are showering or massaging your breasts during feeds.
- Try to empty the affected breast thoroughly at each feeding.
- Use the 3 Fs for treating plugged ducts. Feed baby *First, Frequently*, and *For longer* on the affected side.
- Apply a warm compress (heating pad, hot water bottle or gel pack) to the affected breast or take a warm shower before feeding your baby. This helps unclog the breast.
- While feeding baby, gently massage the breast downward or toward the nipple. This helps to break up and drain the plugged duct.
- If there is still milk in the breast after feeding, use a breast pump or hand express until the breast is thoroughly drained.
- Alternate baby's feeding positions to optimize drainage of all ducts. Try a different position with each feed.
- Alternate the breast you start the feeding with each time.
- Tie a ribbon or place a safety pin on your bra to remind you which breast to start feeding with at the next feed. This is especially helpful for those 3 a.m. feedings.
- Avoid wearing constrictive clothing or underwire nursing bras.
- If you are prone to mastitis, avoid wearing nursing bras to bed or sleeping on your stomach.
- Compressing your breast with a finger (to create an air space for baby's nose) or your hand (to support your breast) during a feed may lead to a duct blockage.
- Keep the nipple clear of any crusting or dried milk. Gently clean your breasts with a soft cloth and warm water (no soap) when necessary.

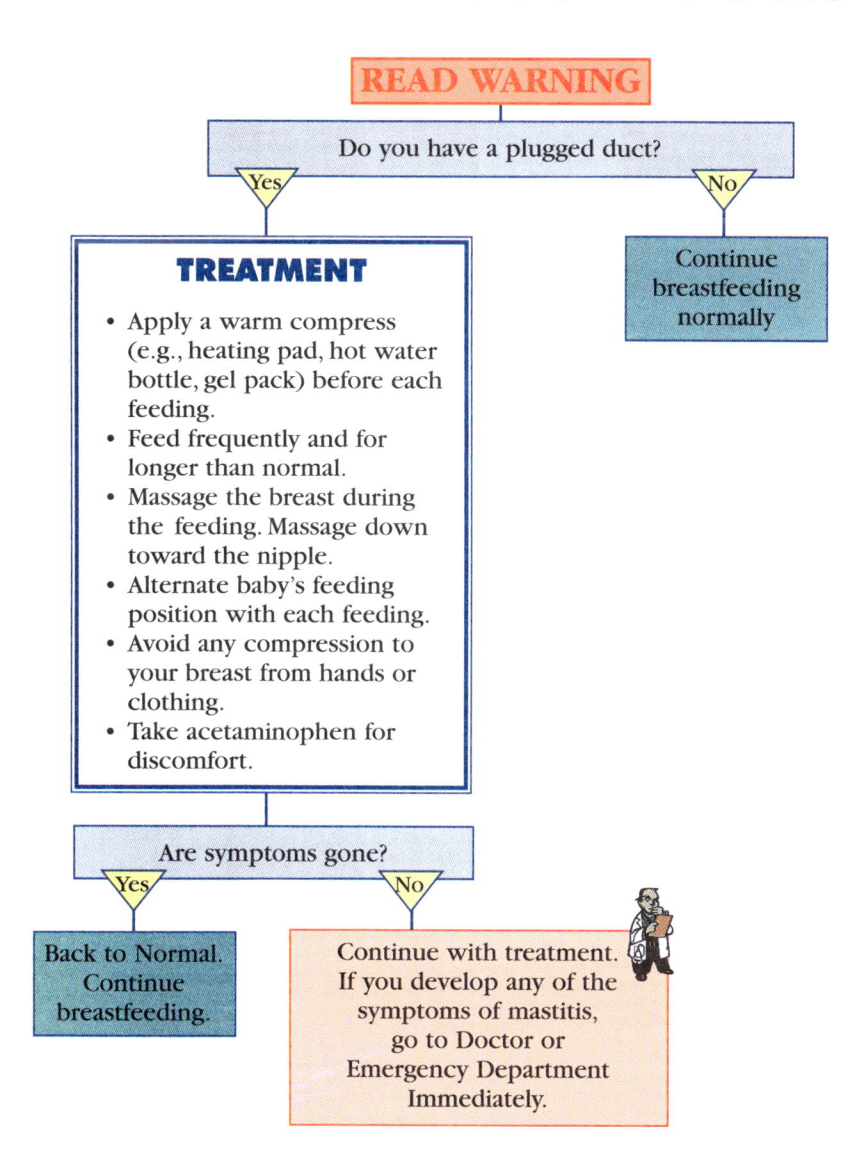

BREAST: PLUGGED DUCTS

READ WARNING

Do you have a plugged duct?

No → Continue breastfeeding normally

Yes ↓

TREATMENT

- Apply a warm compress (e.g., heating pad, hot water bottle, gel pack) before each feeding.
- Feed frequently and for longer than normal.
- Massage the breast during the feeding. Massage down toward the nipple.
- Alternate baby's feeding position with each feeding.
- Avoid any compression to your breast from hands or clothing.
- Take acetaminophen for discomfort.

Are symptoms gone?

Yes → Back to Normal. Continue breastfeeding.

No → Continue with treatment. If you develop any of the symptoms of mastitis, go to Doctor or Emergency Department Immediately.

BREAST: PLUGGED DUCTS

Trade Secrets

- Plugged ducts can occur at any time while you are breastfeeding.
- Plugged ducts normally disappear within 24 to 48 hours when treated correctly.
- Lumps in the breast usually occur when the breast is not being properly drained.
- Don't stop or slow down breastfeeding or you will make the problem worse. Keep going and get helpful advice.
- Having plugged ducts puts you at higher risk for developing a breast infection (mastitis).
- Plugged ducts are best prevented by breastfeeding regularly and keeping the milk flowing!
- Proper latch is crucial for the proper draining of the breasts. If you have any problems speak to your lactation consultant.
- See your lactation (breastfeeding) consultant early and regularly for any breastfeeding problems. This includes any problems starting or maintaining breastfeeding or when considering switching to formula because of problems.
- Most doctors have not been taught the art of breastfeeding.

Definitions

- **Areola** is the colored circular area around the nipple.
- **Mastitis** is an infection of the breast.
- **Plugged ducts** are clogged milk ducts that halt or slow milk flow and often lead to breast infection.

Synonyms

- Blocked ducts • Breast lumps • Caked breasts • Breast plugs

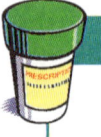

Medications/Treatments

- **Acetaminophen**, with or without codeine, is used to treat pain and fever. Codeine improves pain control.
- **Antibiotics** are used to treat breast infections (e.g., mastitis).
- **Breast massage** during feeding helps to drain the breast and clear plugged ducts.
- **Breast pumping** or **hand expression** help drain breast milk from the breast. See pumping (page 139) and storing milk (page 142).
- **Warm showers** or **compresses** help to encourage milk flow.

BREAST: SORE/CRACKED NIPPLES

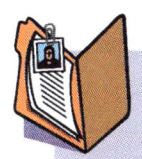

CASE STUDY

Sharon was two days postpartum and had just been discharged from the hospital when I got a call from her.

"My nipples are all cracked and bleeding," she groaned. "My toes curl and I have to hold my breath every time my baby latches. I knew that breastfeeding would take a while to get used to but I'm starting to dread every feeding. Is breastfeeding supposed to hurt this much?"

The home visit examination revealed two cracked and scabbed nipples. The breasts were soft. There was no evidence of mastitis.

Sharon sustained nipple trauma (damaged nipples), which led to sore and cracked nipples.

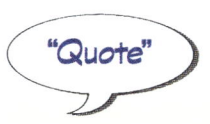

"Quote"

Sore nipples are almost always associated with a poor latch. Fix the latch and the problem fixes itself.

Cracked nipples are a recipe for disaster. Treat them fast so they don't last.

BREAST: SORE/CRACKED NIPPLES

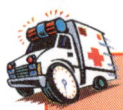

WARNING
Go to your Doctor if you have ANY of the following:
- Cracked or bleeding nipples
- Baby stops feeding or fails to gain adequate weight (5 to 7 oz./week under 4 months of age)
- Baby does not wet or dirty at least six diapers daily
- A skin condition on the nipples (e.g., scaling, rash, oozing, crusting or the nipple turns white, red or shiny)
- A burning pain lasting throughout the feeding • Any signs of mastitis
- It is too painful to breastfeed • The pain continues despite treatment
- Swollen, red or purple nipples

SYMPTOMS
- Burning, throbbing or shooting pain in nipples or breasts
- Cracked, bleeding, blistered nipples that are painful when baby latches

GOALS
To determine the cause of pain.
To treat symptoms to attain a pain-free latch.

TIPS
- Feed baby frequently and always ensure there is a correct latch, so that your breasts do not become too full and, therefore, more difficult for baby to latch on to.
- Vary baby's feeding positions to prevent skin breakdown and to promote better emptying of the breasts.
- Hand express before a feeding so milk is already flowing or "letting down" when you put baby to the breast.
- Feed baby as soon as possible after baby awakens.
- Breast massage during feeding may assist with milk flow.
- When taking baby off your breast (unlatching), insert your finger into the corner of baby's mouth far enough until a popping sound is heard (like breaking a vacuum seal) and take baby quickly away from the breast.
- After feeding, express some breastmilk onto the nipple and air dry or use a hairdryer (on the low setting) to dry your nipples.
- Lanolin-based nipple creams may be helpful. Apply sparingly and do not wash off before the next feeding.
- Wash nipples once daily with water. Avoid all soaps and cleaning products. Do not scrub your breasts or nipples.
- Change breast pads frequently. Choose pads that have no plastic backing. Air dry nipples as much as possible.
- Babies can be very aggressive when sucking. Start with the less sore nipple when baby's sucking is most vigorous and switch to the other nipple when baby's sucking has slowed.

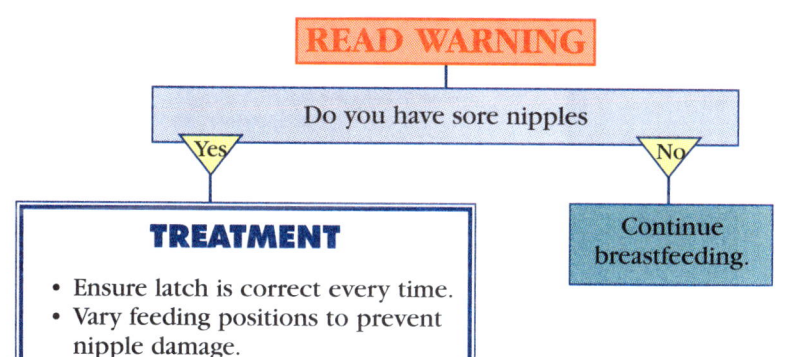

BREAST: SORE/CRACKED NIPPLES

READ WARNING

Do you have sore nipples

Yes →

No → Continue breastfeeding.

TREATMENT

- Ensure latch is correct every time.
- Vary feeding positions to prevent nipple damage.
- Feed baby frequently and early to prevent baby getting over-hungry.
- Get milk flowing before baby latches.
- Avoid breast engorgement.
- Apply expressed breastmilk to nipples after every feed. Allow to air dry.
- Avoid the use of all products on the breast. This includes all creams, oils cleansers, fragrances, soaps, etc.
- Go to a lactation consultant at the first sign of breastfeeding problems.
- Go to your doctor at the first sign of a breast infection.

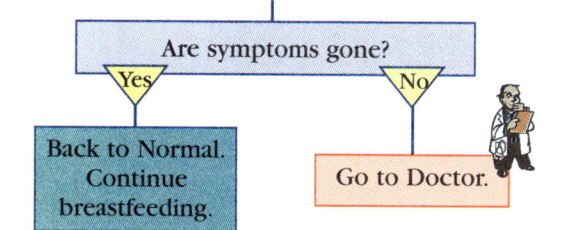

Are symptoms gone?

Yes → Back to Normal. Continue breastfeeding.

No → Go to Doctor.

YOUR HOME DOCTOR™ Mom

BREAST: SORE/CRACKED NIPPLES

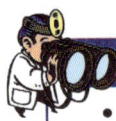

Trade Secrets

- Most nipple soreness is related to a poor latch (see Latching Your Baby, page 130).
- Most women feel some discomfort (but not pain) while breastfeeding is being established.
- Women who have very sensitive skin may be more prone to nipple damage.
- Most nipple discomfort resolves within the first week.
- Some babies are aggressive nursers with an amazing latch and suck. While there is no treatment for this, you must learn to protect your nipples while allowing them to harden naturally.
- Your nipples are naturally protected by oil glands on the areola. These also lubricate the nipple. Cleaning with soaps, alcohol or cleansers removes these natural protective products.
- Anything that will assist in the let down of your milk will make it easier for your baby to suck. Try relaxation techniques or a glass of beer to promote a good let down.
- Beware of pacifiers and bottles, which can lead to "nipple confusion." Using these may cause problems with proper breast latching.
- See your lactation (breastfeeding) consultant early and regularly for any breastfeeding problems. This includes any problems starting or maintaining breastfeeding or when considering switching to formula because of feeding problems.
- Most doctors have not been taught the art of breastfeeding.

Definitions

- **Areola** is the colored circular area around the nipple.
- **Thrush** is a yeast infection of the skin.

Synonyms

- None

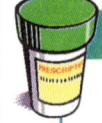

Medications/Treatments

- **Antibiotics** (creams or pills) are used to treat infections.
- **Acetaminophen**, with or without codeine, is used to treat pain and fever. Codeine improves pain control.
- **Lanolin-based nipple creams** provide a nipple moisture barrier and promote healing by preventing drying and scabbing.
- Most commercial and cosmetic products should be avoided.
- **Nipple Shields** are latex or silicone sheaths shaped like a mexican hat and used for sore and inverted nipples.

YOUR HOME DOCTOR™ Mom

CESAREAN SECTION RECOVERY

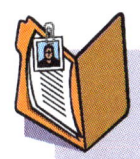

CASE STUDY

I visited Jeanine in hospital the day after her cesarean section.

"Thanks for coming," she said. "I am at a bit of a loss. I have had normal deliveries before and would know what to expect then, but I feel completely out of my element with this C-section. Could you tell me what I should expect in the next few weeks?"

I spent the next 15 minutes answering her questions and concerns and describing how to heal over the next few weeks and months.

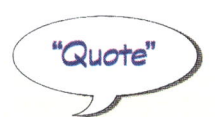

"Quote"

There is no "easy way" to have a baby. Just by making it to the other side of any labor and delivery, you deserve respect, admiration and a cold beer.

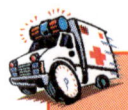

CESAREAN SECTION RECOVERY

WARNING
Go to your Doctor if you have ANY of the following:

- Fever above 38.5°C (101.3°F) • Chills • Dizziness • Sudden chest pain
- Redness, heat, swelling, gaping, discharge or odor at incision site
- Increasing pain • Vaginal blood clots larger than half your palm
- Increasing vaginal flow • Heart rate greater than 100 beats per minute
- Trouble urinating or passing gas • Leg pain or swelling

SYMPTOMS
- Lower abdominal tightness or a pulling sensation

GOALS
To promote a safe and speedy recovery from major surgery and childbirth.

TIPS
- Walk as soon as possible. When walking, try to stand as straight as possible.
- Avoid lifting, carrying or doing housework. Remember, you are recovering from major surgery. You need to be nurtured!
- Breastfeed with good pillow support, or on your side. Have someone hand you and take the baby to allow you to reposition.
- Equip the home with everything for mother and baby on the same floor for at least the first two weeks after recovery.
- Limit the number of visitors, especially during the first month.
- Support your abdomen when you stand, cough, laugh or sneeze.
- At the first sign of an infection, go to your doctor.
- The bowels go to sleep for one or two days after any abdominal surgery. Don't start eating until your bowels start working.
- Enemas or rectal suppositories may help reduce abdominal pain from trapped gas and stool. Walking may also help.
- Cover the incision during the day to prevent rubbing. Leave dressing off at night to air dry the wound (unless it is draining).
- Support your abdomen and be careful what you do. Avoid exercising for at least six weeks after delivery to allow things to heal.
- Gas pains or cramps may last seconds to minutes during the first few days post-surgery. They will resolve when the bowel function returns to normal.
- Drink plenty of fluids to replace your losses.
- Empty your bladder regularly.

CESAREAN SECTION RECOVERY

WHAT TO EXPECT

DAYS 1 – 3:

- You may feel groggy or nauseated from the anesthetic. A spinal or epidural will leave you numb from the abdomen to your feet. Stay in bed for at least 12 hours.
- You may have backaches or headaches after epidurals.
- Your wound will hurt when the anesthetic wears off.
  (Request pain medication when you START to feel the pain.)
- Pain in your shoulder may occur after abdominal surgery.
- Nurses will monitor your recovery and assist with regular dressing and pad changes.
- IV and urine catheter will be removed, usually after 24 hours.
- A switch from needles to pills for pain medication.
- A need for assistance with breastfeeding and childcare.
- An evaluation that bowel and bladder function is restored.
  – Take only fluids at first. (No caffeinated or carbonated drinks.)
  – Start solid food only after you can pass gas from your rectum.
- You may shower 48 hours after surgery.
- Bed rest with a slow, gradual increase in movement usually starting around 8 to 24 hours.

DAYS 4 – 14:

- Staples or stitches are removed. Dissolvable sutures usually disappear by two weeks. The incision may burn or itch as it heals.
- Discharge from the hospital is usually between days 4 and 7.
- A need for assistance with housework and lifting (including baby).
- Acetaminophen, with or without codeine, for pain relief.
- A slow but progressive increase in movement is possible.
- Some difficulty with bowel movements (especially if taking narcotics for pain control).
- Do not lift anything heavier than your baby.
- Get plenty of rest. You will feel fatigued.

WEEKS 2 – 6:

- Lochia disappears but you need to continue iron supplements.
- Minimal discomfort, tightening or stretching pain.
- Continued improvement in strength, flexibility and endurance.
- For sexual intercourse, wait at least four weeks postpartum.
- Your skin may burn, itch or feel numb around the incision site.
- You may feel intermittent pulling sensations under the scar.
- You may start exercising (slowly) once you are pain free.

CESAREAN SECTION RECOVERY

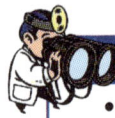

Trade Secrets

- Cesarean section is major abdominal surgery. It may take up to six months for you to make a complete recovery.
- Having a C-section may cause a delay in breastfeeding.
- Scars take at least one year to heal completely. The scar will change from red to pink and fade over this time. Scar numbness may last for months or may never resolve completely. Keep the scar protected from the sun for at least six months for best healing results.
- Exercises to tighten abdominal muscles are most important after a cesarean birth, but wait six weeks before starting.
- It is very important to get moving after having a cesarean section. The sooner you move, the sooner you mend.
- Abdominal pains may be worse after having a cesarean than after a vaginal birth. They should improve over the next six weeks.
- Expect the same postpartum difficulties (except for a lack of vaginal pain) that you would have following a vaginal delivery.

Definitions

- **Cesarean section** is a surgical procedure involving cutting open the uterus and abdominal wall to allow for the delivery of an infant instead of vaginal delivery.
- **General anesthetic** puts you to sleep before surgery.
- **Increased mobilization** means increasing activities and walking.
- **Local anesthetic** (e.g., epidural, spinal) results in loss of pain in a limited area.
- **Lochia** is a vaginal discharge of leftover blood, mucus and tissue from the uterus after delivery.

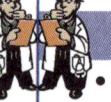

Synonyms

- C-section • Cesarean • Section

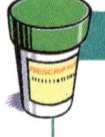

Medications/Treatments

- **Acetaminophen**, with or without codeine, is used for pain relief and fever control.
- **Ice packs** or **warm packs** (gel packs, hot water bottles, heating pads) reduce discomfort and promote healing.
- **Stool softeners** help you have a bowel movement without pain.
- **Abdominal support** with pillows or hands assists with pain relief and helps to prevent wound tearing. Support is especially helpful when coughing, sneezing or laughing. Abdominal girdles are also helpful for abdomen and wound support.
- **Support stockings** are often used after surgery to prevent blood clots and reduce swelling. They improve leg circulation.

CONSTIPATION

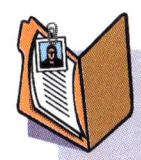

CASE STUDY

Arlene came in to the office for her six week postpartum checkup.

"I thought once I had the baby my constipation problems would be over," she lamented. "I admit that I haven't been eating as well as I was during my pregnancy but I still drink six to eight glasses of water per day. It's just that sometimes I feel too tired to eat, let alone exercise or spend any quality time with my bowels every day."

Examination revealed a healthy but tired new mother. We reviewed the treatment basics for constipation in the postpartum period. We then discussed postpartum survival strategies.

Arlene had constipation. With some minor adjustments she was better within a week.

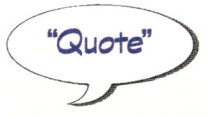

"Quote"

Constipation is our body's way of reminding us to get back to the basics. This means more exercise, vegetables, fruits, fiber and most of all fluids.

Constipation after birth leads to another painful delivery.

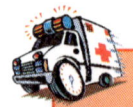

CONSTIPATION

WARNING
Go to your Doctor if you have ANY of the following:

- Severe, constant or worsening abdominal pain
- Fever above 38.5°C (101.3°F) • Rash • Rectal bleeding
- Difficulty passing your stool or urine • Vomiting

SYMPTOMS

- Hard, dry stool that may be infrequent, difficult or painful to pass
- Stomach swelling, bloating and gassiness. Constipation refers to the consistency of the bowel movement, not necessarily the frequency.

GOALS
To recognize and treat symptoms early

TIPS

- Eat frequent small nutritious meals. Do not skip meals.
- Exercise regularly. Moving your muscles helps to move your bowels. Walking is a great choice of exercise.
- Drink six to eight glasses of fluid daily. The best choices are water and diluted juices. Avoid alcohol and caffeinated products.
- Schedule a regular time for your bowels every day. One of the best times is 10 minutes after a meal or coffee. After breakfast is a good choice.
- A warm drink such as tea or hot water with lemon half an hour before breakfast may help to stimulate your bowels.
- Foods to use: Any food with increased fiber or bran such as whole grain breads, cereals, fresh fruits, prunes, vegetables, popcorn, figs, pears, beans. Increase fiber intake slowly to avoid excessive gas production and allow your bowels time to adapt.
- Foods to avoid: Dairy products, caffeine, chocolate, bananas, white rice, apples, toast or foods high in fat or sugar. Reduce high-residue or highly processed foods (most fast foods).
- People sometimes find it easier to pass a stool when their feet are elevated on a footstool while they are sitting on the toilet.
- Add 1 or 2 tablespoons of bran to cereal each morning.
- Check labels for fiber content in foods.
- Take fiber supplements if you are prone to constipation.
- Many medications, pain killers, antidepressants, antacids and herbal and vitamin supplements (especially those with iron) cause constipation.

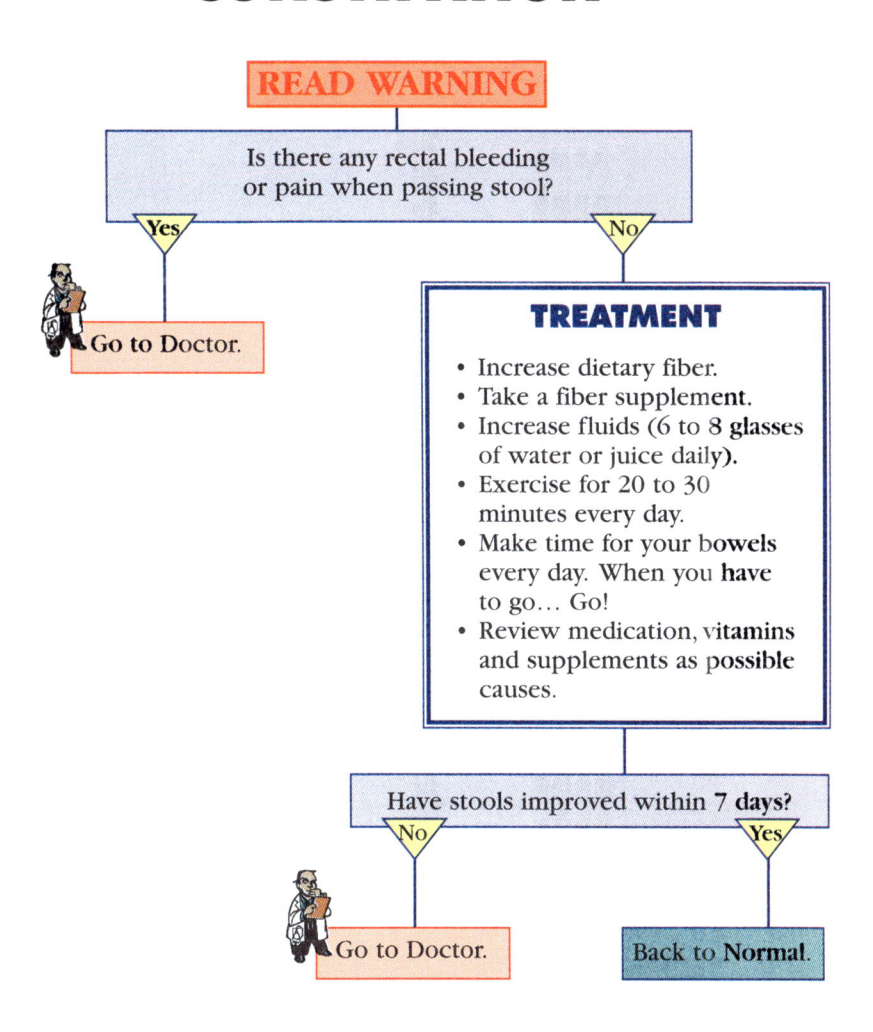

CONSTIPATION

READ WARNING

Is there any rectal bleeding or pain when passing stool?

- **Yes** → Go to Doctor.
- **No** →

TREATMENT

- Increase dietary fiber.
- Take a fiber supplement.
- Increase fluids (6 to 8 glasses of water or juice daily).
- Exercise for 20 to 30 minutes every day.
- Make time for your bowels every day. When you have to go… Go!
- Review medication, vitamins and supplements as possible causes.

Have stools improved within 7 days?

- **No** → Go to Doctor.
- **Yes** → Back to Normal.

Avoid the following:
mineral oils, laxatives, stool softeners or enemas including herbal (naturopathic) remedies without the advice of your doctor.

YOUR HOME DOCTOR™ Mom

CONSTIPATION

Trade Secrets

- Constipation refers to the consistency of the bowel movement, not necessarily the frequency.
- "Normal" bowel movements can range anywhere from three times a day to three times a week.
- Recommended daily dietary fiber intake is 20 to 35 grams. Most people get 10 to 15 grams.
- Increase fiber content in your diet slowly to allow your bowels to adapt.
- Learning good bowel habits means listening to your body.
- Constipation that doesn't go away in a few days may mean a more serious problem. See your doctor without delay.
- Processing and refining foods usually removes fiber. You should eat foods as close to their natural state as possible.

Definitions

- **Anal fissure** is a small crack or tear in the rectum as a result of the passage of a large or hard (constipated) stool.
- **Constipation** is the infrequent passage of hard, dry stool.
- **Enema** is the introduction of a liquid into the rectum to promote clearing of the bowel. This clears the lower part of the bowel from severe constipation.
- **Fiber foods** are those high in roughage (e.g., unmilled bran)
- **Stool** is bowel movement (stool, poo, crap, number 2, feces)

Synonyms

- Bunged up • Plugged up

Medications/Treatments

- **Acetaminophen** may be tried for pain.
- **Saline enemas** are used to flush the lower bowel in severe constipation.
- **Exercise** (see page 69) helps your bowels move.
- **Fiber supplements** add mass to your stool and stimulate the bowel to push things along. You must take these with plenty of fluids to avoid further constipation.
- **Herbal remedies** abound for constipation. Always check with your doctor before using.
- **Hot water bottle, heating pad** or **heating packs** soothe aches and pains.
- **Laxatives** are sometimes tried for severe constipation. Laxatives can be dangerous and habit-forming. Always check with your doctor before using.
- **Suppositories** (e.g., glycerine) are inserted into the rectum to stimulate a bowel movement.

DEPRESSION

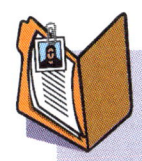

CASE STUDY

Brenda was eight weeks postpartum when she came in to the office with her husband.

"You've got to help Brenda," her husband said. "Ever since the baby was born she has become terribly depressed. She is crying all the time, she isn't eating or sleeping and is becoming paranoid that people are constantly laughing at her."

Brenda agreed that she had started feeling very depressed after the birth of their baby. She was having difficulty with her concentration and energy levels, and was also feeling "trapped" and very emotional, with feelings of anger and sadness. She wasn't eating well and the nighttime feedings had worsened her insomnia to the point where she now hadn't slept for three days. She also admitted that she had the feeling that people were laughing at her weaknesses and attempts at mothering. She was feeling worthless, helpless and hopeless.

Brenda had developed a severe postpartum depression.

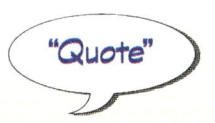

"Quote"

*Depression isn't just feeling bad.
It's a real and serious illness that leaves you
feeling out of control of your own emotions!*

*Feeling worthless, helpless, hopeless?
Then seek out help for mental illness.*

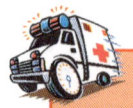

DEPRESSION

WARNING
Go to your Doctor if you have ANY of the following:

- Uncontrolled mood fluctuations
- Feelings that you want to harm yourself or someone else (including your baby)
- Severe feelings of rejection • Becoming withdrawn • Nightmares
- Feeling out of control • Thoughts of suicide

SYMPTOMS
- Depressed mood • Crying spells • Poor concentration
- Loss of interest in doing things you previously enjoyed (including sex)
- Feeling anxious or exhausted • Difficulty falling or staying asleep
- Uncontrolled mood fluctuations
- Feeling out of control, helpless, hopeless, worthless, rejected or inadequate

GOALS
To recognize the signs of depression and seek treatment early.

TIPS

- Maintain open, honest communication between partners.
- Reassurance and support for mom is of utmost importance.
- Build a support network of friends, family or other community supports including experienced moms.
- Discuss feelings of inadequacy, stress, uncertainty, anxiety or guilt or your dreams with your family, friends or doctor.
- Get out every day and do something active. Go for a walk.
- Fears and conflicting feelings about parenting are common.
- Balance your life with work, rest, family and exercise.
- Ask for help. Accept help. Get dressed every day.
- Keep a journal or diary. Write down how you feel. List three good things that happen to you each day.
- Drug therapy is usually necessary in moderate to severe cases of depression.
- Drug therapy combined with psychotherapy is most helpful.
- Check with your doctor before starting any medicines. This includes any over-the-counter or herbal or vitamin therapies.
- Light therapy works well for some seasonal depressions.
- Get help with your new baby. Hire someone if necessary.
- Depression is common after any stressful life transition. Babies are definitely a life transition and can be very stressful.
- Avoid all alcohol and recreational drugs.
- Do not skip meals. Eat frequent small nutritious snacks.
- Avoid high-sugar and high-fat junk foods.
- Try relaxation techniques, tai chi, yoga, meditation or prayer.

DEPRESSION

READ WARNING

Emotional Symptoms Possible in Postpartum Depression

- Depressed mood
- Anger
- Anxiety
- Guilt
- Loss of interest in things
- Loss of control
- Loss of confidence
- Feeling helpless, hopeless and worthless
- Poor concentration
- Frequent crying spells
- Feeling overwhelmed
- Thoughts of hurting yourself (suicidal)
- Thoughts of hurting baby or others
- Confusion
- Agitation and irritability
- Inability to enjoy yourself
- Overly sensitive
- Low self-esteem
- Trouble making decisions

Physical Symptoms Possible in Postpartum Depression

- Loss of energy
- Headaches
- Loss of appetite or overeating
- Change in weight
- Fatigue/loss of energy
- Food cravings (sugar/starch)
- Excessive sleeping
- Trouble falling asleep or staying asleep
- Hot flashes or chills
- Anxiety or panic attacks
- Nausea and vomiting
- Trouble breathing (shortness of breath)
- Heart palpitations or racing heart
- Increased sweating
- Tremors or shakiness
- Backaches

Are you experiencing any of these symptoms of depression?

Yes → Go to Doctor Immediately.

No → Normal.

Always take suicide thoughts and threats seriously!

YOUR HOME DOCTOR™ Mom

DEPRESSION

Trade Secrets

- Depression occurs in up to 20% of all mothers.
- It may occur any time within the first six months after delivery.
- Postpartum depression symptoms often worsen if: the mother or infant are unwell, the mother is experiencing marital difficulties, there is excessive stress related to home and/or work or if children are closely spaced or if the mother lacks adequate social support.
- Postpartum "blues" is different from depression. It usually starts within three days of delivery and lasts less than two weeks.
- Go to your doctor if your symptoms are severe, last longer than two weeks or prevent you from doing normal activities.
- Postpartum "blues" becomes postpartum depression when you feel so bad that you cannot function in your everyday life.
- Depression is always worsened by lack of sleep. Take a nap.
- Friends and family should always take threats of suicide seriously.

Definitions

- **Anxiety** is a troubled or uneasy state of mind.
- **Depression** is an illness that includes feelings of dismally low spirits with associated emotional and physical symptoms.
- **Fatigue** is an overwhelming tiredness.
- **Fears** are an excess in agitation and anxiety caused by the expectation or the realization of danger.
- **Mood swings** (emotional lability) are fluctuations in emotions.
- **Paranoid** is a mental disorder with delusions of persecution.
- **Stress** is physical, mental and emotional strain resulting from adapting to the changing demands of life.

Synonyms

- Depressed • Downhearted • Feeling Blue • Melancholy

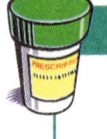

Medications/Treatments

- **Antidepressant medications** are used to treat depression. They take two to six weeks to work, so the sooner you see your doctor the sooner you will start to feel better.
- **Anxiolytic (anti-anxiety) medications** are used to treat feelings of anxiety as well as anxiety or panic attacks.
- **Exercise** may be helpful in the treatment of depression.
- **Psychotherapy** (counseling) is talk therapy. It is good for mild depression and in combination with drug therapy for moderate to severe depression.
- **Light therapy** is effective for depressions worsened by lack of exposure to sunlight. This is especially common in northern latitudes.

EMOTIONS

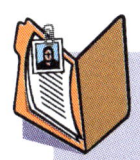

CASE STUDY

Kendra was four weeks postpartum when she came into the office.

"I feel like I'm an emotional wreck," she exclaimed. "The first week I was feeling euphoric and happy, last week I was feeling anxious and overwhelmed, and now I am feeling angry and depressed. Some days my emotions even change from minute to minute. My husband says it's like living with someone on an emotional roller-coaster. How can I get off this ride?"

The physical examination was normal. We spent the rest of the visit discussing normal emotional responses to pregnancy, birth and the postpartum period.

Kendra was reassured when she discovered that she was normal and not going crazy.

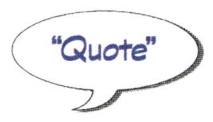

"Quote"

Anxiety is a state of apprehension and psychic tension – a state of mind common to all parents.

Parenting isn't all glamour. It is hard work, dedication, sleep deprivation and anxiety interspersed with frequent periods of heart-bursting joy.

*I love being a mother...
I am more aware. I feel things on a deeper level.
I have a kind of understanding about my body,
about being a woman.* - Shelly Long

EMOTIONS

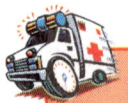

WARNING
Go to your Doctor if you have ANY of the following:

- Feelings of anxiety or depression • Severe feelings of rejection or isolation
- Loss of interest in usual activities • Uncontrolled mood fluctuations
- Feeling out of control or that you want to harm yourself or others (including your baby) • Difficulty going to or staying asleep
- Using drugs or alcohol to help you cope

SYMPTOMS

- Feeling elated, anxious, nervous, tearful, stressed, tense, inadequate, guilty, resentful, angry, overwhelmed, tired, oversensitive, lonely, helpless or sad
- Poor sleep, appetite or concentration. Go to your doctor immediately if any of these symptoms are severe, prolonged (more than two weeks) or stop you from doing your normal activities.

GOALS

To deal with emotions and develop your support network.

TIPS

- Dreams and conflicting feelings about parenthood, including anxiety and inadequacy, are common and normal.
- Emotions and mood swings are best managed by talking about them. Discussion is the foundation of emotional care.
- Build a support network of friends, family, community resources and other mothers. Learn not to compete.
- Parenting is the one profession where there is no apprenticeship or degree. You are boss from day one. This responsibility is best met with an observing eye, an open mind and a passion to learn.
- Strive for a balanced lifestyle including work, family, exercise and rest. Remember to keep some time for yourself every day.
- Take care of your own physical needs. Eat frequent small nutritious snacks throughout the day.
- Get out of the house every day, especially on bad days. Take your baby to the park, mall or a mother support group.
- Use your phone as your link to the outside world. Set up a support network of new moms. Talk to at least one adult every day.
- Getting sleep is vital. Without it your coping strategies will fail. That's why sleep deprivation is used as a form of torture.
- Develop and rely on your parents' intuition. Trust your instincts.
- A baby's life (especially in the first few months) is very unstructured. Changes in daily routine are not failures.
- Don't expect too much of yourself too early. Let yourself grow.
- Try to find an element of humor even during disaster days.

EMOTIONS

READ WARNING

Do you feel any of these common emotional changes or symptoms?

- Mood swings/emotional lability • euphoria/excitement/joy
- uneasiness/anxiety/fear/doubt • depression/crying
- **feeling** inadequate/overwhelmed/difficulty adapting to motherhood
- low energy/fatigue • diminished memory or concentration

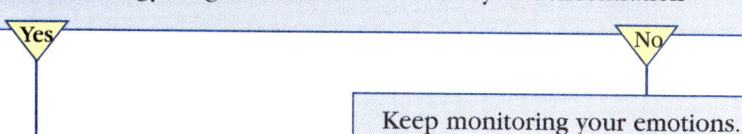

Yes / **No**

No → Keep monitoring your emotions.

TREATMENT
Suggested Providers of Emotional Support

- **Sp**ouse or partner
- **M**other, mother-in-law or close relative
- **A fr**iend or neighbor who is also a mom
- **D**evelop a mentor (someone to model yourself after)
- **J**oin mother support organizations
- **P**ublic health, private nurses, midwives
- **C**ounseling or hospital services.
  (Hospital warmlines or nurse call-in support centers)
- **Y**our family doctor
- **Y**our religious leader
- **B**ooks on parenting

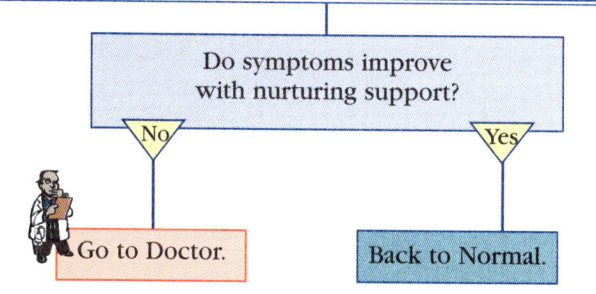

Do symptoms improve with nurturing support?

No → Go to Doctor.

Yes → Back to Normal.

Acknowledge your achievements, however small, every day. Congratulate yourself!

YOUR HOME DOCTOR™ Mom

EMOTIONS

Trade Secrets

- More than 50% of new mothers experience the blues.
- The blues normally start two to seven days after delivery and resolves without medical treatment within two weeks.
- The trick in dealing with the normal emotional changes of motherhood is knowing that you are not alone. Most women feel the same way. Talk, talk, talk to resolve concerns.
- Parenthood is one of the biggest life changes that you and your partner will ever deal with. Don't be afraid to ask for help.
- Your doctor should be your foundation of support and advice during this turbulent time. When booking an appointment for baby, make sure you book time to discuss your concerns too.
- Women are often expected to transform themselves into mothers simply by the biological act of giving birth. This is an impossible expectation. Learn your new role together with your baby, set small achievable goals and remain flexible to change.
- Be kind to yourself, and always keep your sense of humor.

Definitions

- **Anxiety** is a troubled or uneasy feeling or state of mind.
- **Depression** is an illness that includes the feeling of dismally low spirits with associated emotional and physical symptoms.
- **Fatigue** is an overwhelming tiredness.
- **Fears** are an excess in agitation and anxiety caused by the expectation or the realization of danger.
- **Mood swings** (emotional lability) are fluctuations in emotions.
- **Stress** is physical, mental and emotional strain resulting from adapting to the changing demands of life.

Synonyms

- Moods • Feelings • Sentiment • Attitude • Sensitivity • Sensitive

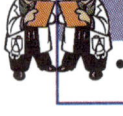

Medications/Treatments

- **Antidepressant medications** are usually used to treat moderate to severe cases of depression.
- **Anxiolytic (anti-anxiety) medications** are used to treat anxiety.
- **Exercise** helps promote physical and emotional comfort after delivery. Feeling healthy and good about your body helps in the emotional recovery.
- **Psychotherapy** (counseling) is used to deal with psychological difficulties. This includes emotional problems.
- **Relaxation therapy** (through art, meditation, tai chi, yoga, prayer, etc.) assists in the control of emotions.

EPISIOTOMY/PERINEAL PAIN

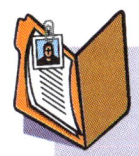

CASE STUDY

Isabelle was one week postpartum when she came in to the office.

"I don't know what to blame," she said. "Between my 10 pound baby, the forcep delivery and the episiotomy, I can't believe how sore I am. All I know is it hurts like hell to sit down. Just to add to my concern, I started getting a slight vaginal discharge yesterday. I just had to come in and make sure that everything was okay and will hopefully improve in the next few days."

On examination, the episiotomy was clean and healing well. The vaginal exam revealed a normal postpartum vaginal discharge. The vaginal swelling was just starting to settle and there were no vaginal tears. The uterus was already shrinking back to a normal size.

I reassured Isabelle that all was on the mend. We discussed the importance of daily sitz baths. I also explained to her that as the stitches dissolved she might develop a slight increase in vaginal discharge. I reiterated that if at any time she was concerned, or if the discharge changed she should be rechecked.

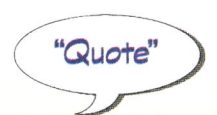

"Quote"

And in time this too shall pass...

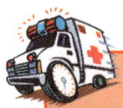

EPISIOTOMY/PERINEAL PAIN

WARNING
Go to your Doctor if you have ANY of the following:
- Dizziness or light headedness • Fever above 38.5°C (101.3°F)
- Pain that is worsening or preventing sleep • Chills
- A sudden increase in vaginal bleeding • Malodorous discharge
- Difficulty passing urine or stool
- Pus, redness, heat or a gaping incision site

SYMPTOMS
- Vaginal pain due to tearing or from surgical cuts (episiotomies) performed during a vaginal delivery • May feel more uncomfortable with sitting, throbbing when standing and makes intercourse impossible

GOALS
To minimize pain and improve mobility

TIPS
- Sitz baths (soaking your bottom in lukewarm water) provide comfort and promote healing. Sitting on a vinyl inflatable donut also relieves the pressure on your bottom.
- Try lying flat, with your stomach supported with a pillow.
- Wash your hands well both before and after changing sanitary pads or after going to the washroom.
- Ice packs are helpful in reducing pain and swelling.
- Use a doctor-recommended pain killer.
- Avoid constipation by eating fruit and fiber and drinking plenty of fluids.
- Start gentle pelvic floor exercises (Kegels) as soon as possible. Increasing the frequency and duration daily.
- Chilled witch hazel, salt water and antiseptic solutions have shown no specific healing benefits over cleansing with lukewarm water. Use whatever gives the most soothing comfort.
- Try baby wipes for cleaning yourself after using the toilet.
- Wear a sanitary pad to absorb any vaginal discharge. Change these frequently to prevent infection.
- Wear loose, comfortable clothes that promote air circulation.
- Wear cotton underwear for better air circulation and comfort.
- If experiencing pain when passing urine, get checked for an infection. Urinating into the bathwater or sitz bath water may help with the pain. Change the water each time.
- Straddling the toilet when passing urine may help prevent urine coming in contact with tender, healing vaginal tissues.
- Avoid bubble baths, feminine hygiene sprays, deodorant panty liners and pads. Avoid tampon use for the first six weeks.
- Resume sex once you feel comfortable. Vaginal lubrication will likely be needed for intercourse the first few times.

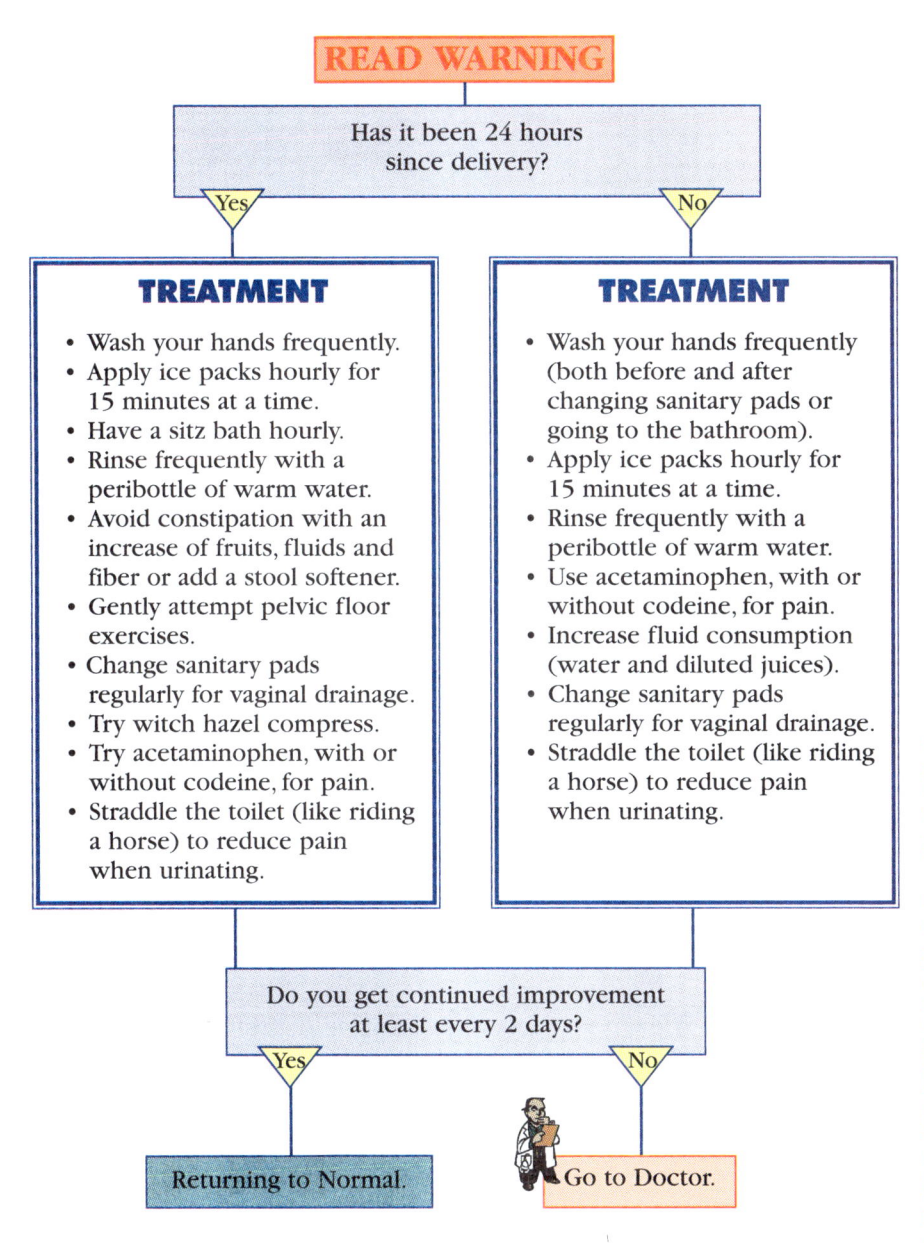

EPISIOTOMY/PERINEAL PAIN

READ WARNING

Has it been 24 hours since delivery?

Yes → TREATMENT

- Wash your hands frequently.
- Apply ice packs hourly for 15 minutes at a time.
- Have a sitz bath hourly.
- Rinse frequently with a peribottle of warm water.
- Avoid constipation with an increase of fruits, fluids and fiber or add a stool softener.
- Gently attempt pelvic floor exercises.
- Change sanitary pads regularly for vaginal drainage.
- Try witch hazel compress.
- Try acetaminophen, with or without codeine, for pain.
- Straddle the toilet (like riding a horse) to reduce pain when urinating.

No → TREATMENT

- Wash your hands frequently (both before and after changing sanitary pads or going to the bathroom).
- Apply ice packs hourly for 15 minutes at a time.
- Rinse frequently with a peribottle of warm water.
- Use acetaminophen, with or without codeine, for pain.
- Increase fluid consumption (water and diluted juices).
- Change sanitary pads regularly for vaginal drainage.
- Straddle the toilet (like riding a horse) to reduce pain when urinating.

Do you get continued improvement at least every 2 days?

Yes → Returning to Normal.

No → Go to Doctor.

EPISIOTOMY/PERINEAL PAIN

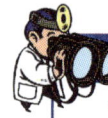

Trade Secrets

- The current trend in medicine is to do fewer episiotomies and only when absolutely necessary.
- Sutures usually dissolve within six weeks. This will depend upon the type of suture material used.
- The speed of healing varies with the extent of tissue damage. Healing is normally completed within one to two weeks.
- Whereas most episiotomies are largely healed by six weeks, pain can last up to nine months in rare cases. Infection and a tear into the rectum are important determinants of healing time.
- The first two weeks are the most painful. Every two days should result in an improvement in discomfort.
- Discomfort with intercourse (sex) may last up to six months.

Definitions

- **Dyspareunia** means painful intercourse.
- **Episiotomy** is an incision, by the doctor, of the external female genital organs used to assist in the delivery of a baby. There are two kinds mid-line and medio-lateral.
- **Peribottle** is a spray water bottle that cleans the perineal area.
- **Perineal pain** is pain at the vaginal opening (actually the area between the vagina and the rectum).
- **Sitz bath** is a lukewarm shallow bath to clean and promote healing of perineal tears and episiotomies.
- **Sutures** are stitches used to sew together vaginal tissue.
- **Vaginal discharge** is any drainage from the vagina. If malodorous, it has a bad smell.

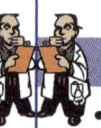

Synonyms

- Episiotomy: 1st degree, 2nd degree or 3rd degree tear
- Suture line • Surgical cut • Surgical incision
- Perineal pain: • Groin pain • Pelvic pain

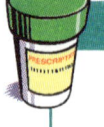

Medications/Treatments

- **Analgesics** are medications for pain control. Acetaminophen, with or without codeine, is one type of analgesic.
- **Exercising** the pelvic floor muscles helps tighten them back to normal to regain support of the uterus, bowels and bladder.
- **Fiber supplements** (psyllium) bulk and soften stool.
- **Ice packs** reduce swelling and control pain.
- **Witch hazel** is a herbal solution that provides soothing relief for perineal pain and swelling.

EXERCISE AFTER DELIVERY

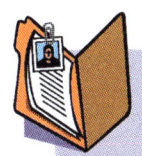

CASE STUDY

Florence came in for her six week postpartum checkup.

"When can I start getting back to my exercise routine?" she inquired. "I read in a book that it is usually okay to start back around six weeks after delivery, is that correct?"

Her exam showed normal healing.

We discussed the start-low (short periods of time) go-slow (gradual increase in intensity and duration) approach to resuming her exercise routine, meaning that you start with easy, gentle exercises and progress slowly back to your desired exercise level. In this way stretching and strengthening of the muscles can be attained without risk of injury.

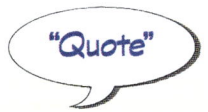

"Quote"

In resuming exercise after the stress of having a baby, remembering to "Start-low and go-slow" is most important.

Exercise your mind, body and spirit just for the health of it.

EXERCISE AFTER DELIVERY

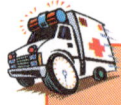

> **WARNING**
>
> *Go to your Doctor if you have ANY of the following:*
>
> - Chest pain • Racing heart • Trouble breathing
> - Severe headaches, dizziness, light-headedness or blurred vision
> - Fainting spells • Blurred vision
> - Back, pelvic or abdominal pain or cramps • An increase in vaginal bleeding
> - Pain, swelling or redness in the leg

GOALS

To regain strength, flexibility and endurance.

TIPS

- Exercise with your baby. Start by going for walks together.
- Make a commitment! Start today. You only need about 30 to 60 minutes of light to moderate exercise or 20 to 30 minutes of vigorous exercise each and every day.
- Listen to your body. No pain, no gain is not the axiom to follow after delivery. If it hurts, don't do it. Work to the level you feel comfortable at. Be realistic in your goals.
- You should be able to carry on a normal conversation when exercising. If you can't, slow down!
- Monitor your aerobic exercise with a target heart rate chart.
- Good hydration is vital when exercising. Consume about 1 liter (1 quart) of water for every hour of aerobic activity.
- Wear comfortable, loose-fitting clothing. Wear a supportive sport or nursing bra and purchase comfortable and supportive exercise footwear. Don't wear a girdle during exercise.
- When breastfeeding, time your exercise routines right after feedings.
- Wear two well-fitted sports bras at the same time to support lactating breasts. This will provide added support and comfort.
- A five-minute warm-up should precede all exercise.
- Aerobic exercise can be done three to five times a week starting with 15-minute to 30-minute intervals. Muscle stretching and strengthening can be performed up to three times a week.
- Avoid jerky and bouncy movements.
- Pelvic floor exercises (Kegels) should be done every day and as many times a day as humanly possible.
- Join a fitness club if possible. This will provide exercise, important social contacts and motivation.
- Alternatively, try exercise tapes or television exercise programs.
- Aerobic exercises that elevate your pulse to 75% of maximum are best. (220 minus your age, multiplied by .75 gives you this 75% of maximum target heart rate.)

EXERCISE AFTER DELIVERY
POSTURE

Maintaining good posture in everything you do will help you **recover** after delivery and prevent injuries.

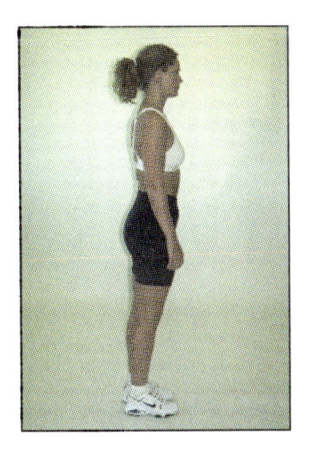

1. Stand - without slouching

2. Sit - without slouching

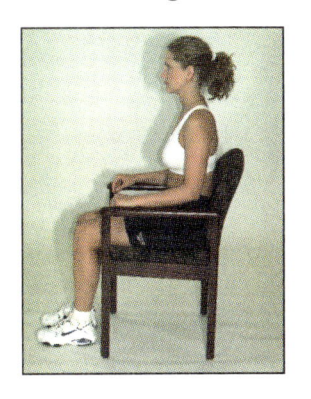

3. When lying down
    - support your body.

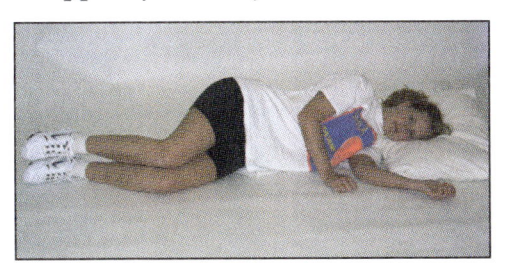

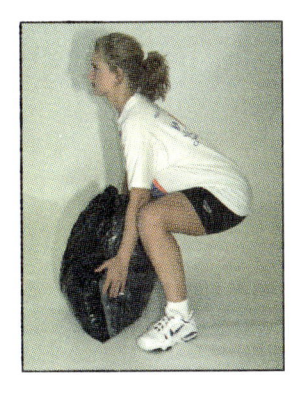

4. When lifting small bundles
    - bend your knees.

YOUR HOME DOCTOR™ Mom   71

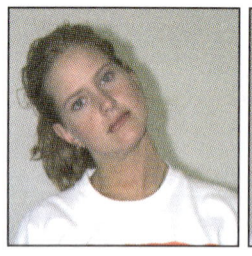

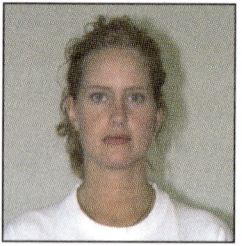

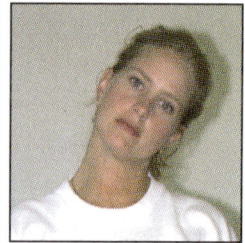

EXERCISE AFTER DELIVERY

BREATHING

Breathing right is as important as exercising right. Always breathe in when relaxing muscles and breathe out when tightening muscles. Never hold your breath during exercise. Try to breathe in slowly through your nose while expanding your stomach. Then breathe out through your mouth. Time breathing in should match time breathing out.

WARM-UPS AND COOL-DOWNS

Warm-up and cool-down exercises usually include range of motion exercises to prepare and repair muscles for endurance and strength activities. See the flexibility (stretching) routine below. Take at least 10 minutes to warm-up before and cool-down after any exercise routine.

EXERCISING

FLEXIBILITY (Range of Motion Exercises)

These exercises are designed to help stretch your muscles and joints. Try to avoid bouncing when stretching as your joints and ligaments are still unstable. Use slow, steady movements and don't stretch to your maximum for the first several weeks. Hold each movement for 15 to 20 seconds. Breathe slowly in through your nose and out through your mouth. Tai chi and yoga are also excellent flexibility exercises.

Stretching from top to bottom

Neck – Range of motion exercises

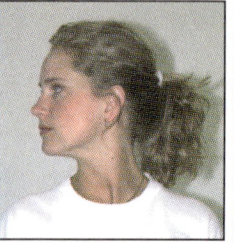

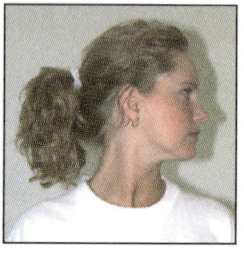

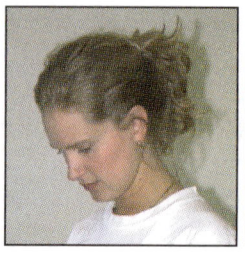

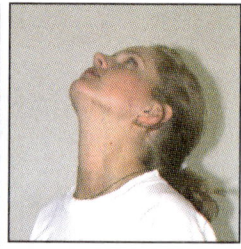

EXERCISE AFTER DELIVERY
FLEXIBILITY

Chest – Stick em up stretch

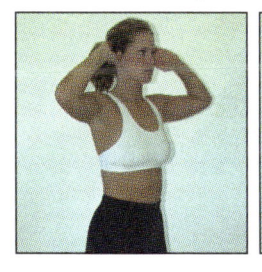

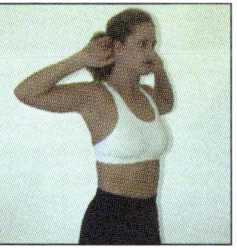

Hips – Hula stretch

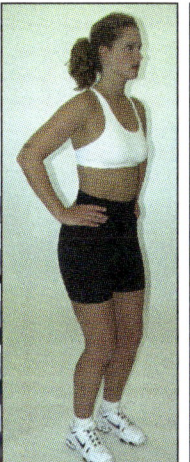

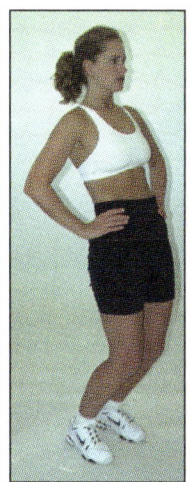

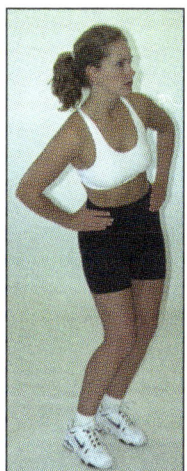

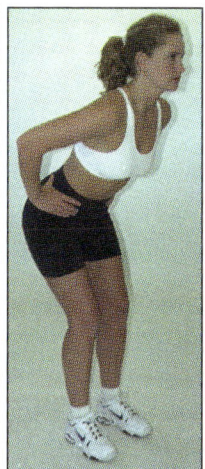

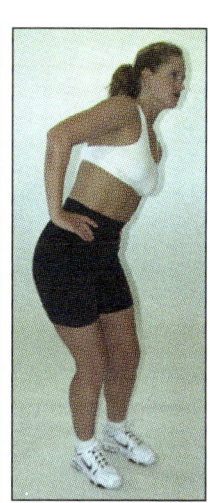

Inner thigh stretch and Quad strengthening – Horse riding stretch

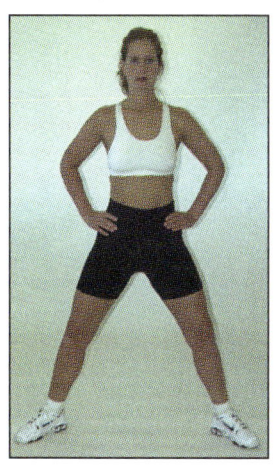

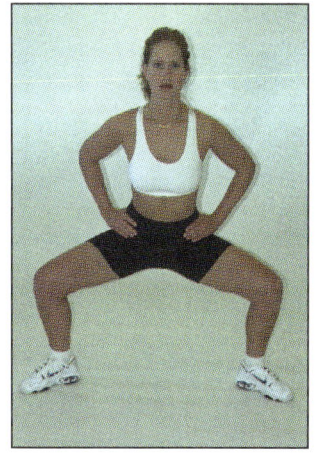

EXERCISE AFTER DELIVERY
FLEXIBILITY

Hamstrings and Calves – Bottoms up. Do right, then left.

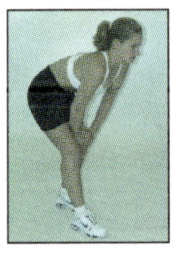

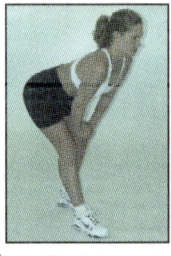

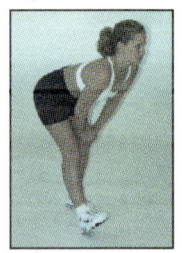

Hips and Inner Thighs – Sprinters stretch. Do right, then left.

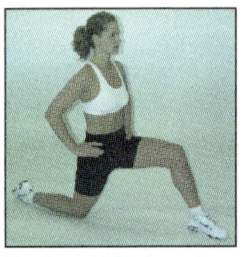

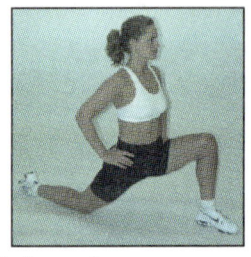

Back and Thighs – Praise God stretch

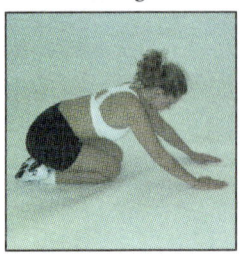

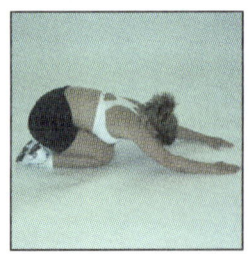

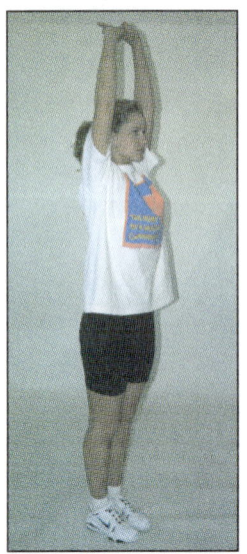

Cleansing Breath –
Reach for the sky stretch to finish.
Remember to breathe in through your nose and out through your mouth.

EXERCISE AFTER DELIVERY

ENDURANCE (Aerobic Exercises)

These exercises are specifically for your heart and lungs. They help you stay healthy, prevent diseases and help provide more energy in your everyday activities. Examples include walking, swimming, jogging, biking, rollerblading, cross-country skiing, skating, rowing, dancing, aerobics, skipping, hiking. Do not exceed your target heart rate.

> *Vigorous exercise may cause a build up of lactic acid in breastmilk. This makes the milk taste bad for baby, so breastfeed before and one to two hours after vigorous exercise routines.*

STRENGTH (Strengthening Exercises)

These exercises help keep your bones and muscles strong. They help recondition muscles after delivery. A pound of fat burns about 4 to 7 calories a day, whereas a pound of lean muscle burns about six times that amount! You must check for a diastasis recti before starting abdominal exercises. See your doctor first. Do all the following strengthening exercises in a slow and controlled motion. Water bottle exercises (or tin cans or books) may be used in place of free weights for strengthening.

Neck – Press head firmly against hand and hold for 10 to 15 seconds.

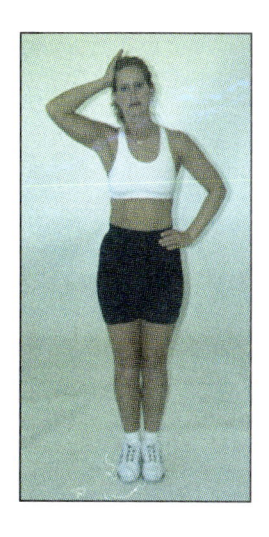

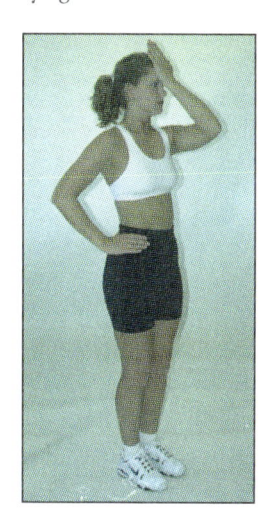

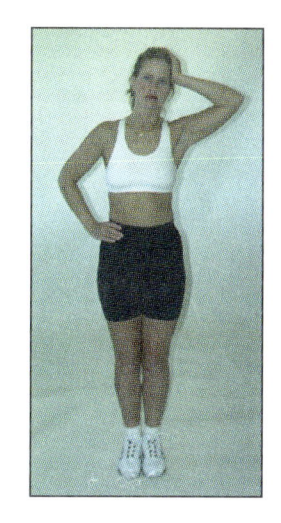

EXERCISE AFTER DELIVERY
STRENGTH continued

Shoulders – Side raise. With your arms straight, raise your hands (with water bottle) to shoulder height. Repeat 10 to 15 times.

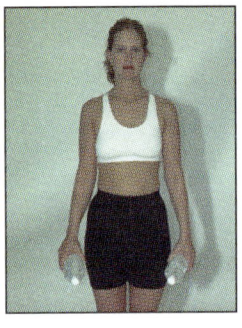

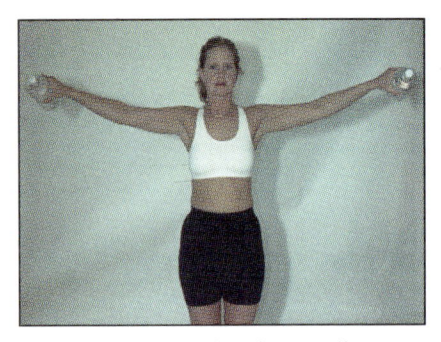

Arms – Bicep curl. With palms facing forward and your elbows at your side, raise your hand toward your shoulder. Repeat 10 to 15 times.

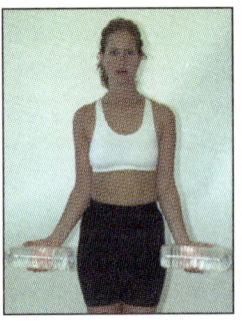

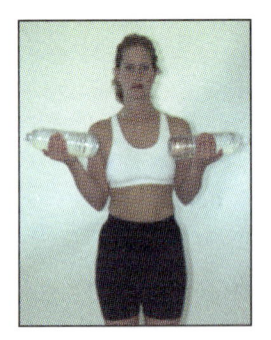

Arms – Tricep kick-back. Hold on to the back of a chair. Bend over, and keep the other arm parallel to the floor. Straighten the arm behind you. Repeat 10 to 15 times.

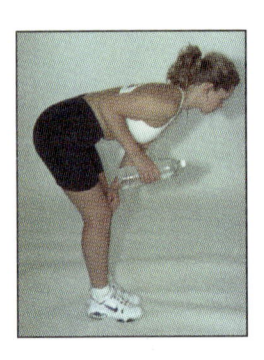

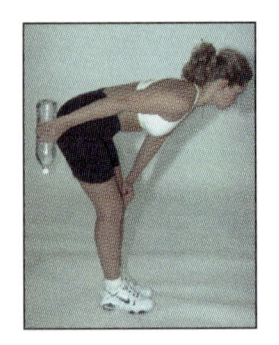

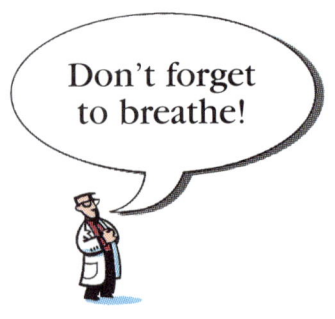

Don't forget to breathe!

EXERCISE AFTER DELIVERY
STRENGTH continued

Back – Bent over row. Hold on to the back of a chair. Bend over, and extend your hand toward the floor. Raise your elbow until your hand touches your breast. Repeat 10 to 15 times.

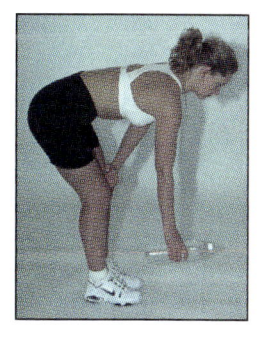

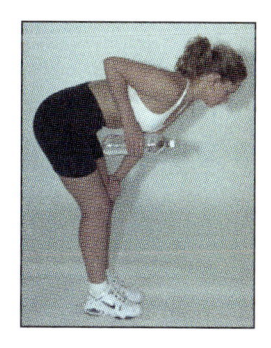

Hips and Buttocks – Leg raise. Stand with one foot on the stair. Move the other leg forward then back. Do not arch your back.

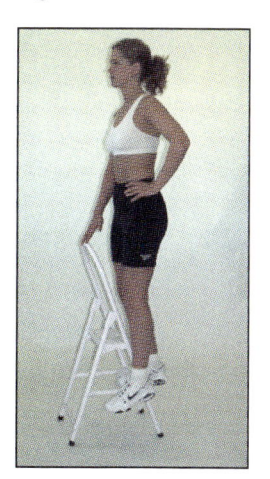

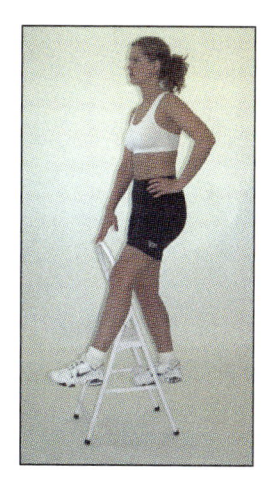

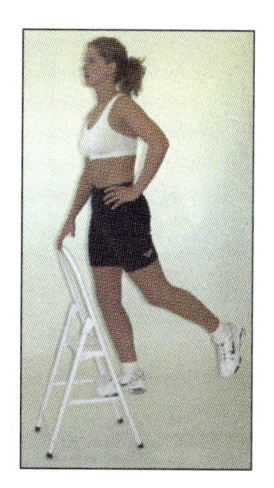

Chest – Pushup. Keep your hands in line with your shoulders and wide apart. Do not arch your back. You can also do this exercise while standing up and pushing against the wall.

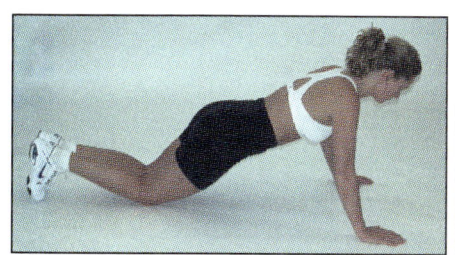

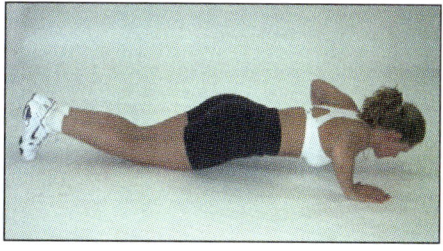

EXERCISE AFTER DELIVERY
STRENGTH continued

Abdominal area–Cross-overs. Lie on your back with your knees bent. Tilt your knees to the right, then to the left. Do each side 10 to 15 times.

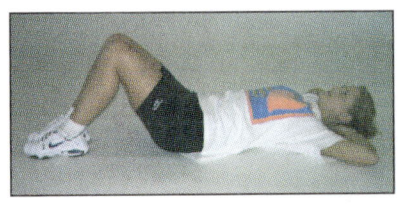

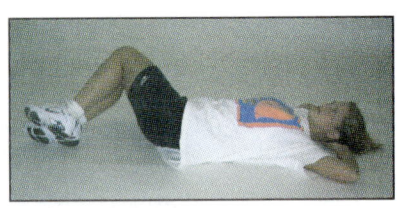

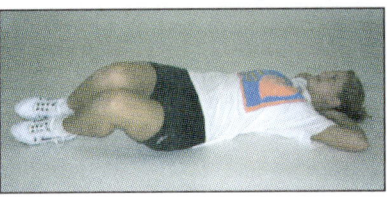

Abdominal area–Dead bug. Lie on your back with your knees bent. Place arms over head. Raise your right knee and right arm toward each other. Keep knee bent and head on the floor. Repeat 10 to 15 times. Repeat on the left side.

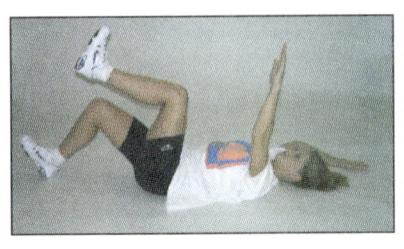

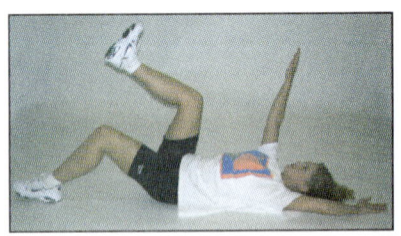

Lower back–Extensions. Lie on your stomach with your hands above your head. Raise your right hand and left foot 6 to 8 inches (15 to 20 centimeters). Repeat 10 to 15 times. Repeat with left hand and right foot. Keep your head on the floor throughout.

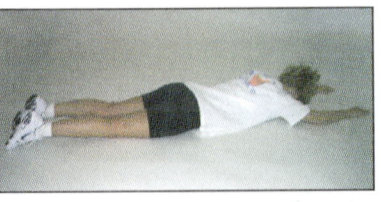

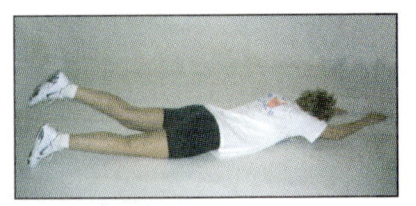

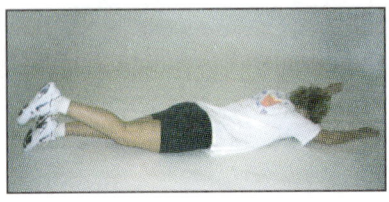

EXERCISE AFTER DELIVERY
STRENGTH continued

Lower abdominals–Pelvic tilt (this exercise can be done sitting, standing or lying down). The goal of this exercise is to squeeze your tummy muscles to remove the arch in the lower back.

Standing pelvic tilt.

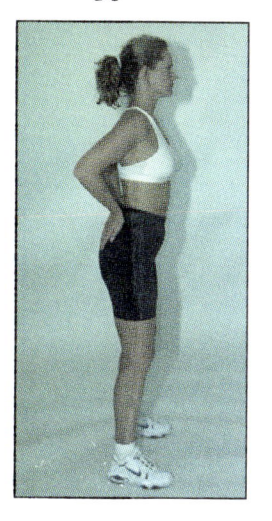

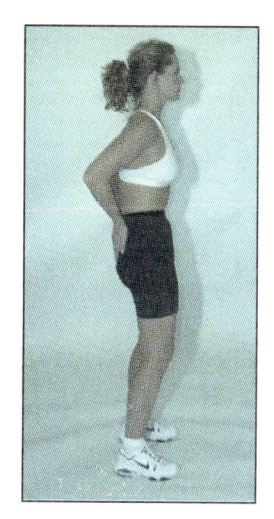

Lying pelvic tilt.

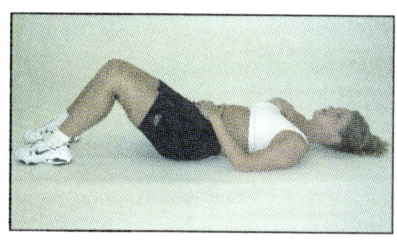

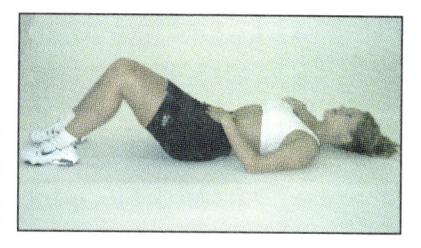

> **Pelvic floor** – Kegel exercises. Kegels are the most important exercise to heal traumatized perineal muscles. You must first learn to isolate each of the muscle groups. Lie on your back with knees bent and feet shoulder-width apart. Squeeze the rectum as if you were trying to stop from passing gas. Then squeeze the vagina as if to prevent losing a tampon. Then squeeze as if you were trying to stop yourself urinating. While squeezing count from 1 to 10 and then 10 to 1. Repeat 5 times. Increase the frequency and duration of your Kegels as tolerated.

EXERCISE AFTER DELIVERY

Trade Secrets

- Exercise after delivery is important for physical and emotional health. It also helps recondition your traumatized body.
- Speak with your doctor before restarting any exercise program, especially after a traumatic birth or cesarean section.
- Have your doctor check you for diastasis recti (splaying of your abdominal muscles). Specific abdominal exercises will be needed to prevent hernias if you have this condition.
- Exercise is most easily done as a family thing. Enjoy your new baby as you exercise together. Do exercises with your baby or place baby in a position where they can watch you. They love it.
- Plan exercise into your daily schedule. Challenge yourself.
- Making a commitment to your health will help to keep you healthier for others as well. Start a plan, then plan to start.
- Try a new physical activity such as tai chi or yoga. Many sport clubs have a free trial period. Some even have babysitting.
- Start slow, with just a few and very deliberate toning exercises, and build gradually, both frequency and duration, as you progress.
- Exercising a small amount every day or several times a day is the best way to encourage weight loss and improve your tone.
- Remember, athletic parents produce athletic children.

Definitions

- **Aerobic exercise** is exercise to improve heart and lung conditioning. It improves circulation and oxygen uptake throughout the body. It is important for weight reduction.
- **Diastasis recti** is the separation of the rectus abdominus muscles running down the center of the abdomen as a result of stretching during pregnancy or delivery.
- **Exercise** is the exertion of body and mind to condition and improve one's health.

Synonyms

- Exercising • Fitness • Toning • Working out

Medications/Treatments

- **Exercise** comes in a variety of flavors. Find one you like so that you can continue exercising for the long run.
- Have your partner **massage** your tired, sore muscles at the end of the day.

FATIGUE (TIREDNESS)

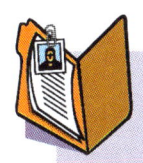

CASE STUDY

Marilyn came in to the office one afternoon. She was twelve weeks postpartum.

"I can't believe how tired I am," she groaned. "Between the nighttime feedings, household chores and organizing my husband and two older kids, I hardly have enough time to scratch myself. This week work called up to see when I would be returning to my position at the bank. I am so tired all the time. When will I get my energy back? Do you think I'm getting postpartum depression?"

Examination revealed a tired but otherwise healthy mother. We arranged some blood tests, which later revealed a mild case of anemia (low iron). Further discussion did not uncover any of the symptoms of postpartum depression.

Marilyn had fatigue.

We discussed possible solutions to her very busy life and started her on iron supplements and vitamins.

By her next visit Marilyn was feeling much more in control and much less fatigued. Her family had started helping out more around the house. She had even returned to her work outside the home.

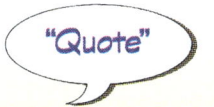

"Quote"

Fatigue in the postpartum period is inversely proportional to the amount of sleep and directly proportional to the household demands.

All mothers are "working mothers."

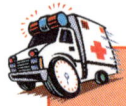

FATIGUE (TIREDNESS)

WARNING
Go to your Doctor if you have ANY of the following:

- Pale skin • Excessive tiredness/fatigue • Fainting or dizzy spells
- Heart palpitations • Chest pain • Difficulty breathing (shortness of breath)
- Symptoms of depression: feeling hopeless, helpless or worthless; crying spells; poor concentration; loss of interest in usual activities; severe mood fluctuations; difficulty going to sleep or staying asleep; feeling out of control; feeling you want to harm yourself or someone else

SYMPTOMS
- Excessive tiredness due to new demands on your body, mind and emotions • Sleep deprivation

GOALS
To get enough rest to deal with normal daily requirements.

TIPS
- Establish your priorities. (Hint: Baby and you.)
- Establish your goals for the day. Keep them reasonable.
- Make lists for everything. Do the most important things first.
- Eat a well-balanced diet with proper intake of iron, protein, fluids, vegetables and fruit. (See Nutrition, page 97.) Eat frequent small meals and snacks. This is called grazing. Choose foods that are high-fiber and low-fat. Avoid fast foods.
- Foods rich in iron include red meats, beans, peas, nuts, prunes, lentils, whole wheat breads and green leafy vegetables.
- Take your vitamins. Maternal vitamins after delivery are okay.
- Rest whenever possible, sleep whenever practical.
- Listen to your body. Alternate activity with short rest periods.
- Sleep when your baby sleeps. Take a "power nap."
- Exercise to help relieve fatigue (but avoid overdoing it).
- Go to bed an hour earlier and get up half an hour later.
- Ask a friend or family member to "borrow" your older children for part of a day so you can have some rest and recovery time.
- Improve efficiency to reduce work. Group your work tasks.
- Always accept help from others when offered.
- Have your doctor check for medical causes of tiredness (anemia/low iron) if fatigue persists.
- Speak with your family about how best to share the workload.
- See your doctor at the first sign of depression.
- Say no to things that will add stress and cause more fatigue.
- Stop smoking. Limit your alcohol and caffeine intake.
- Exercise your sense of humor daily. The stronger your sense of humour is, the stronger you are.

FATIGUE (TIREDNESS)

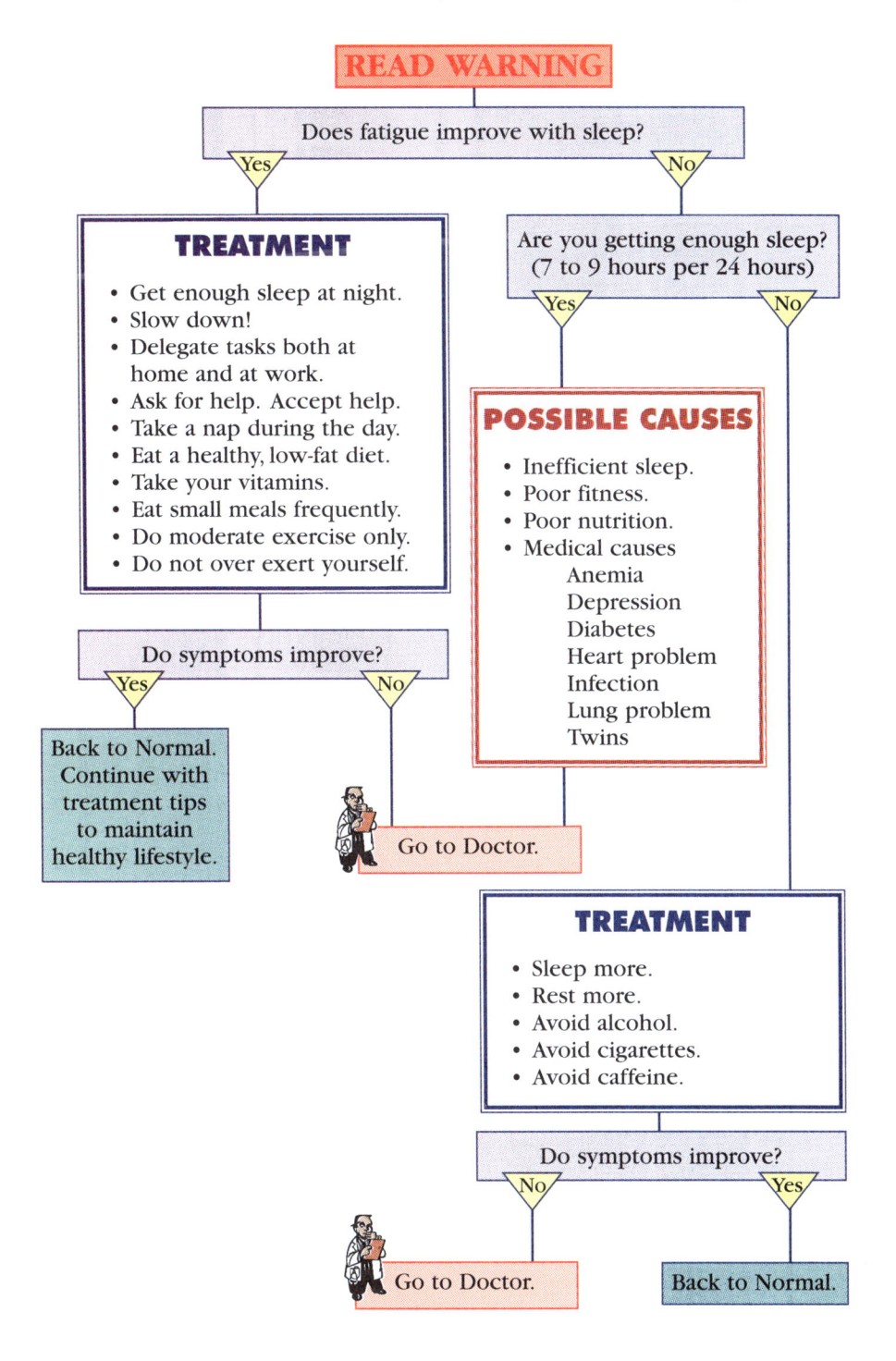

READ WARNING

Does fatigue improve with sleep?

Yes →

TREATMENT

- Get enough sleep at night.
- Slow down!
- Delegate tasks both at home and at work.
- Ask for help. Accept help.
- Take a nap during the day.
- Eat a healthy, low-fat diet.
- Take your vitamins.
- Eat small meals frequently.
- Do moderate exercise only.
- Do not over exert yourself.

Do symptoms improve?

Yes: Back to Normal. Continue with treatment tips to maintain healthy lifestyle.

No: Go to Doctor.

No → Are you getting enough sleep? (7 to 9 hours per 24 hours)

Yes:

POSSIBLE CAUSES

- Inefficient sleep.
- Poor fitness.
- Poor nutrition.
- Medical causes
    - Anemia
    - Depression
    - Diabetes
    - Heart problem
    - Infection
    - Lung problem
    - Twins

Go to Doctor.

No:

TREATMENT

- Sleep more.
- Rest more.
- Avoid alcohol.
- Avoid cigarettes.
- Avoid caffeine.

Do symptoms improve?

No: Go to Doctor.

Yes: Back to Normal.

YOUR HOME DOCTOR™ Mom

FATIGUE (TIREDNESS)

Trade Secrets

- Overdoing it is a common problem. Accept help with home and work commitments from partner, friends and family.
- The secret to surviving fatigue is to weather the storm. If the storm doesn't let up, look for other causes. See the doctor.
- Breastfeeding increases demands on the body. Natural changes in your hormones and metabolism may also cause tiredness.
- Tiredness is from not only lack of sleep but the heightened emotional demands of being a mother.
- Sleep deprivation is a form of torture. Unfortunately, it is also a frequent visitor during the first year postpartum.
- Humans sleep approximately 7 to 9 hours per 24 hours.
- The type of sleep is as important as the amount. REM (dream sleep) is necessary to make you feel both rested and alert.
- Lack of sleep leads to lack of patience. What you need is time to recover with sleep and understanding.
- Try some inspirational music to help you perk up and keep you going. Sing along–your baby will love it!
- Beware of medications. Many can cause fatigue.

Definitions

- **Fatigue** is an overwhelming tiredness as a result of physical, mental and emotional demands.
- **Stress** is physical, mental and emotional strain resulting from adaptation to the changing demands of life. It causes irritability, edginess, stomach upset, headaches, neck or back aches, increased perspiration and rapid breathing and heart rate.
- **Depression** is an illness due to depletion of certain chemicals in the brain. It has a number of symptoms (see the Warning box).

Synonyms

- Drained • Exhaustion • Loss of energy • Tiredness
- Weariness • Weary • Worn down • Worn out

Medications/Treatments

- **Exercise** (see page 69) may help with energy and physical and emotional comfort. Start low, go slow.
- **Nutrition** is important to provide the building blocks for your daily energy demands. Choose high-fiber low-fat foods.
- **Relaxation** techniques or deep breathing exercises may help.
- **Sleep**, whether at night or naps, is vital to improve fatigue.
- **Tai chi or yoga** may help improve your energy levels after delivery.
- **Vitamins** including minerals and iron help to treat tiredness.

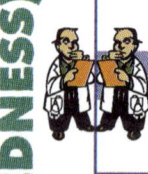

HEMORRHOIDS

CASE STUDY

Mariah was sixteen weeks postpartum when she came to the office.

"These darn hemorrhoids are driving me crazy," she stated. "They cause me more discomfort than the episiotomy did. I thought once I delivered they would go away and leave me alone. Instead, I'm having as much trouble now with itching, bleeding and soreness as I did in my last trimester of pregnancy. I've tried all the treatments I used during my pregnancy but nothing seems to be helping. Doc, do you have any magic to make them disappear?"

On examination Mariah had two large blue hemorrhoids. They were swollen, sore and bled with the slightest pressure.

Mariah had developed postpartum hemorrhoids. One of them was thrombosed (had developed a blood clot within it) and had to be surgically drained.

"Quote"

Think of them as varicose veins of your bottom with a mean streak.

Remember, the sooner you treat, the sooner you'll sleep.

HEMORRHOIDS

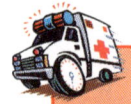

WARNING

Go to your Doctor if you have ANY of the following:
- Painful hemorrhoids • Blood or pus in the stool
- Other sites of bruising or bleeding • Sudden change in bowel movements
- Difficulty passing bowel movements • Passing black, tarry stools
- Pain that doesn't improve with treatment
- Hemorrhoids that cannot be pushed back into the rectum
- Fever above 38.5°C (101.3°F)

SYMPTOMS

- Swollen, itchy or painful vein-like pouches of the anus or rectum
- External hemorrhoids may be felt at the anus opening, whereas internal ones usually cannot.

GOALS

To reduce discomfort and swelling and promote healing.

TIPS

- Drink more fluids. Drink six to eight 8-ounce glasses of water a day.
- Increase vegetables, fruit and fiber in the diet. This includes fresh fruit, raw and cooked vegetables, whole grain breads and cereals, prunes, raisins, popcorn, figs, pears and beans.
- Avoid caffeine, alcohol and spicy, acidic or constipating foods.
- Practice Kegel exercises daily (see Exercises, page 79).
- Your goal is to pass a soft, regular bowel movement every day.
- Do not strain when having a bowel movement.
- Schedule time for your bowels every day. The best time is often after a meal, especially breakfast.
- Clean well after each bowel movement. Try warm water on white toilet paper (non-colored and non-perfumed), moisturized tissues, baby wipes or medicated Tucks pads (never soap), and pat dry. Do not rub or wipe when drying your anus.
- Gently push the hemorrhoids back inside after each bowel movement. Then apply some petroleum jelly to the area.
- Apply ice packs to area as often as necessary.
- Soak in a bath of three or four inches of lukewarm water twice a day (Sitz bath). Add a teaspoon of epsom salts to the water.
- Use zinc sulphate hemorrhoid creams or ointments twice a day.
- Go for a walk, or do some form of exercise, every day.
- Apply chilled witch hazel to hemorrhoids to relieve and reduce external hemorrhoid swelling.
- Rest during the day. Lie on your left side to rest and sleep.
- Sit on a donut cushion. Most pharmacies sell these.
- Avoid using laxatives, which can aggravate the problem.

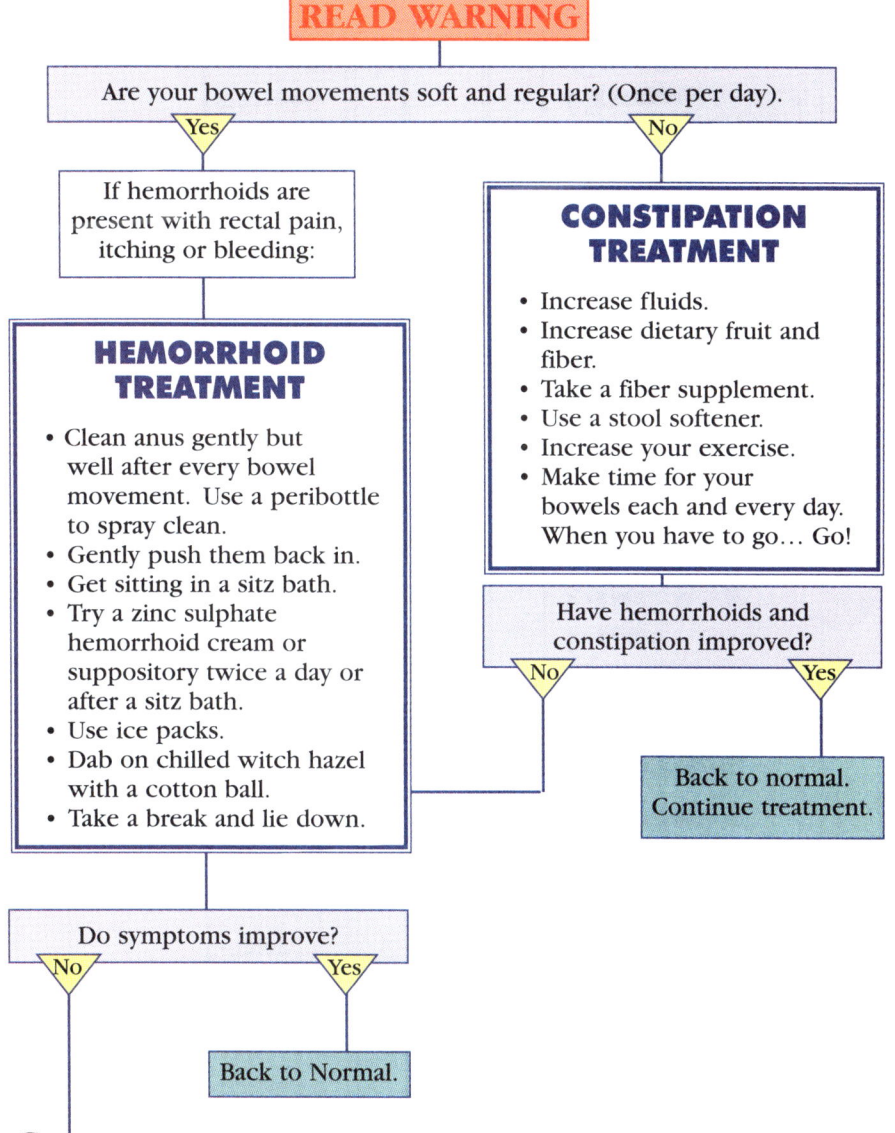

HEMORRHOIDS

READ WARNING

Are your bowel movements soft and regular? (Once per day).

Yes → If hemorrhoids are present with rectal pain, itching or bleeding:

No →

CONSTIPATION TREATMENT

- Increase fluids.
- Increase dietary fruit and fiber.
- Take a fiber supplement.
- Use a stool softener.
- Increase your exercise.
- Make time for your bowels each and every day. When you have to go… Go!

HEMORRHOID TREATMENT

- Clean anus gently but well after every bowel movement. Use a peribottle to spray clean.
- Gently push them back in.
- Get sitting in a sitz bath.
- Try a zinc sulphate hemorrhoid cream or suppository twice a day or after a sitz bath.
- Use ice packs.
- Dab on chilled witch hazel with a cotton ball.
- Take a break and lie down.

Have hemorrhoids and constipation improved?

No → (back to Hemorrhoid Treatment)
Yes → Back to normal. Continue treatment.

Do symptoms improve?

No → Go to Doctor.
Yes → Back to Normal.

YOUR HOME DOCTOR™ Mom

HEMORRHOIDS

Trade Secrets

- Treating constipation well, prevents hemorrhoids swell.
- Hemorrhoids without symptoms require no treatment.
- Any increase in abdominal pressure can lead to hemorrhoids. This includes coughing, sneezing, constipation, laughing, excessive weight gain, tight clothing, lifting, carrying, prolonged sitting, or a baby in your uterus.
- To prevent gas, cramping and diarrhea, always add fiber to your diet slowly. It generally takes about two weeks for your bowels to get used to an increase in fiber content.
- Hemorrhoids during pregnancy often settle with delivery.
- Hemorrhoids often run in families. Ask your mother.
- Mucus is sometimes discharged from hemorrhoids.
- Keep the area immaculately clean to prevent itching.
- Hemorrhoid creams with hydrocortisone (HC) are excellent best for relieving symptoms and shrinking hemorrhoids.
- Creams and ointments may work better than suppositories.

Definitions

- **Anus** is the opening where stool leaves the body.
- **Fiber foods** are those high in roughage (e.g., unmilled bran).
- **Hemorrhoids** are swollen vein-like pouches in the anus.
- **Rectum** is the pouch of bowel above the anus that stores stool before it is passed from the body.
- **Stool** is a bowel movement (stool, shit, poo, crap, number 2).

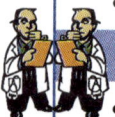

Synonyms

- Piles • "Roids" • Anal grapes

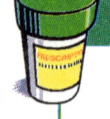

Medications/Treatments

- **Banding** (rubber band ligation) is used to tie hemorrhoids off.
- **Fiber supplements** add fiber to the diet. Fiber supplements and stool softeners help soften stool and soothe bowels.
- **Hemorrhoid creams** help reduce hemorrhoid pain and swelling.
- **Sclerotherapy** is the injection of a solution into hemorrhoids to promote shrinkage.
- **Ice packs** help shrink swelling and reduce the size of veins.
- **Laser, infrared light** and **electrocoagulation** have been used to shrink or destroy hemorrhoids.
- **Medicated Tucks pads** are medicated cleansing pads used for cleaning the anus.
- **Sitz baths** are warm saltwater soaks to help relieve swelling and pain.
- **Surgery** is sometimes necessary to drain a thrombosed hemorrhoid or to treat recurrent hemorrhoids.

MOTHERHOOD (SURVIVAL STRATEGIES)

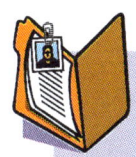

CASE STUDY

Gail returned to the office for the one-year check of her baby Brendon.

"I just want to thank you for all the support, advice and reassurance you gave to me during the past year," she said as I was examining her baby. "Before Brendon, I was a total career professional. I loved my job and never thought anything would change that. I can't believe all the changes that this child has brought to my life. I still love my job but it certainly has taken a back seat to my baby. Who would have thought this could happen to me, the big tough corporate executive? Now I'm working part-time three days a week and spending two days at home with Brendon. My life has improved, but the chaos quotient has definitely increased. Being there for his first smile, sit and walk has made it all worthwhile," she explained. "I was such a novice at this mothering thing, I really had no idea what to do or how to do it, but I wouldn't have missed it for the world."

"I'm really glad that I could help," I responded. "And your thanks has made my day."

"Quote"

To learn about the duality of love and sacrifice, watch and listen to a mother.

Being a mother is learning that chaos can be worn like a badge of honor. When you look around to find things too organized you will sadly find the cause has left home.

MOTHERHOOD (SURVIVAL STRATEGIES)

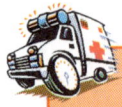

WARNING
Go to your Doctor if you have ANY of the following:

- Concerns that you are failing • Trouble coping
- Feeling depressed, angry or overwhelmed • Feeling out of control
- Thoughts of hurting yourself or the baby
- You keep trying to be supermom

GOALS
To promote physical, emotional and spiritual health for both you and your child.

TIPS

- Becoming a mother can be both exciting and frightening. Suddenly you are faced with new challenges and must make important decisions about a new dependent life.
- You may develop a feeling of being let down or disappointed after the delivery. The perception of constant bliss, the perfect baby and of an adoring family flocking to help is often idealistic and unlikely to happen. This book is your reality guide to common mother concerns.
- Infant demands often lead to maternal fatigue. This fatigue is compounded when mom forgets to tend to her own needs.
- Lack of sleep, lack of support and social isolation can lead to frustration or feeling down. New mothers often feel overwhelmed during this period of readjustment to their new demands.
- New mothers constantly need to re-evaluate priorities and try to maintain a balance between sleep, recreation and work.
- Eat a well-balanced diet. Return to exercise as soon as possible.
- Do you feel guilty about the lack of time or interest in your partner? If so, reassure them that this is just an adjustment phase to a new situation and is only temporary.
- Changes from the pre-baby relationship are often difficult on couples. Make time to communicate concerns and schedule time together as a couple each week.
- Mothers also need time for themselves. This may be a bath at the end of the day or 30 minutes to read a magazine. Always take a few minutes every day for a "sanity break."
- Isolation is a frequent problem for mothers, especially in the first few months after delivery. You must try to get out of the house every day even if only for a stroller walk with baby.

MOTHERHOOD (SURVIVAL STRATEGIES)

TIPS

- To survive, you sometimes have to just let some things go. Don't be an overachiever. Remember, the health of you and your baby comes first. Everything else can wait.
- Many mothers attempt to breastfeed and are unable to do so for a long period or choose to bottle feed from the start. Although breastfeeding has been shown to be the best start for children, being unable to do so for personal or physical reasons does not make you a bad mother.
- Society does not provide adequate support to breastfeeding mothers. It also places high expectations on them to succeed. Avoid feelings of guilt and inadequacy, and seek professional breastfeeding help at the first sign of difficulties.
- New parents often doubt their ability to be a good parent when friends and family are giving their "professional" "what worked for me" advice. Choose two mothers whom you will accept advice from. For all the others, smile, nod and ignore.
- Societal expectations and the desire to be the "perfect mother" often contribute to parents' decreased self-esteem and feelings of inadequacy. Learn to trust yourself and your instincts.
- It is normal for mothers to question themselves about whether or not the choices they make are the right ones.
- Find reliable babysitters early. Make a list and guard it well, as they are worth their weight in gold.
- Alternatively, enjoy time out with other people who also have young kids and bring the kids along. Children travel easily, and taking them along is sometimes less stressful to new parents.
- Be kind to yourself. In parenting, doing your best is always good enough.
- Learn to be an aware and prepared mother. This means knowing what to expect at each development stage and being prepared for the common medical problems possible for each.
- Develop and trust your parents' intuition. Parents usually know when something is wrong with their child. Listen to your inner voice and refuse to be swayed from your concerns.
- Being a mother means learning to live with compromise. This means that new priorities will need to be developed to help you care for both your family and yourself. This means you may have to relinquish some control. No supermoms allowed.
- Learn to ask for and accept help and to learn the art of delegating.
- Try to keep contact with friends and co-workers with quick phone calls every few weeks. Have one adult conversation every day even if this means calling someone up.
- Lack of spontaneity comes with the turf. You will need to develop "organized spontaneity."

MOTHERHOOD (SURVIVAL STRATEGIES)

Trade Secrets

- Seize the moment. Housework will always be there but special moments with your children should be embraced.
- Your life is going to change. This change may be for the better or worse. Learn to anticipate and enjoy change.
- The relationship with your parents will change. Make it something to bind you. Use motherhood to encourage discussion and memories and to make you closer.
- Your relationship with your husband will change. Allow yourself time to slip into your new role as mother and wife. Learn to balance these two important roles without allowing one to dominate the other.
- Get out of the house every day.
- Get involved in an infant/parent program. This is a great way to meet new people with similar interests (babies) and forge new friendships.
- Seek out things that will enhance your child's life. By doing so you will learn to see life, again, through a child's eyes!
- Learn to be organized but flexible. Go with the flow; every day will be different. Things that worked yesterday may fail today.
- Patience is a skill that you will need to practice to perfection.
- Develop your mothering support network early. This includes reliable babysitters, baby-friendly businesses, mother-tot programs, trusted family doctors, your mentor mothers, etc. This will be an evolving document.
- You cannot care for others if you do not care for yourself. This means proper nutrition (no skipping meals!), exercise and rest. It also means time for self and your partner. Work will fill in all the rest of the spaces.
- Keep things simple. Don't complicate child raising.

"NO-TIME" MANAGEMENT

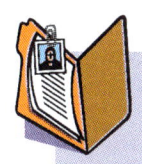

CASE STUDY

Majora was eight weeks postpartum with her first child when I ran into her at the supermarket checkout.

"How's it going at home with the new baby?" I asked innocently.

Majora immediately burst into tears, and we spent the next 20 minutes discussing the profound changes in her life adapting from corporate lawyer to mother. This incredibly professional, organized and proficient attorney felt completely overwhelmed with the new and unexpected demands of a baby with colic.

"I'm having trouble getting organized enough to even get showered and dressed each day," she lamented. "How in the world am I going to be able to get on top of things enough to enjoy my baby, let alone return to work in two months?"

As we talked, I passed on some of the motherhood and "no-time" management tips that I had acquired over the years from other moms.

When I saw her again in the office one week later, things were already starting to improve for both her and baby.

"Quote"

No one gives us time.
We must seek it out then use it efficiently and effectively.

Cleaning your house while your children are still growing is like shoveling the walk before it stops snowing.
— Phyllis Diller

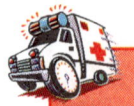

"NO-TIME" MANAGEMENT

> **WARNING**
> *Go to your Doctor if you have ANY of the following:*
>
> - Feeling out of control, isolated or depressed (see Depression, page 57)
> - Feeling that you can't cope • Developing physical symptoms: headaches, chest pain, shortness of breath, dizziness, nausea and vomiting, diarrhea, heart racing or skipping beats.

GOALS

To develop an efficient system of coping with the rigorous demands of motherhood so you won't miss out on the fun.

TIPS

- Determine what is the most valuable use of your time–and do it.
- Make you and your baby a top priority. Demote the importance of housekeeping (especially in the first months).
- Plan to do things as early as you can during the day.
- Do what fills your heart and mind with inspiration.
- Accept offers of help, whether cooking, cleaning, running messages, babysitting, etc. Avoid the superwoman syndrome!
- Buy frozen dinners and casseroles to save time. Prepare frozen meals before delivery if you can.
- Do a large shopping trip before the baby is born. Stock up on everything you could possibly need so you are not running out to the grocery store during the first couple of weeks.
- Stockpile beverages and healthy snacks to use while breastfeeding.
- Prepare baby's room before delivery. Have baby's clothes washed and prepared, and stock up on diapers, wipes, etc.
- Always buy two packs of diapers at a time unless your child is in transition between two sizes.
- Keep diaper supplies on every floor of the house during the newborn stage. It is usual to change diapers 10 to 12 times a day.
- Throw in a load of laundry before bed every night.
- Update the baby journal while waiting at the doctor's office.
- Buy a baby swing and front carrier (baby pouch/sling). They are lifesavers. You can even do housework while using them.
- Run several errands on the same trip. Make a list of everything you wish to accomplish on each errand.
- Develop your support network early on. Rely on them.
- Include your baby in regular "everyday" things that you do, such as getting dressed, putting on make-up, making meals and working out. Babies love to watch mom exercise. Dads do too.
- Be sure to care for your needs as well as baby's.
- Teach your children early on that mom's needs count too.

"NO-TIME" MANAGEMENT

TIPS

- Learn how to leave work unfinished when necessary.
- Learn to Drop, Delay and Delegate (the three D's).
  - Drop things not truly important to do.
  - Delay things that are of lower priority. They can wait.
  - Delegate responsibilities, at home and at work.
- Build breaks into every day. This includes child breaks (where you spend time with your child) and adult breaks (where you spend time with your partner or by yourself).
- Make a space for yourself somewhere in the house that is only for you. Whether a special chair, your bed or a hammock in the garden, let everyone know this is your space when needed.
- Learn to set consistent bedtimes for older children.
- With children, unexpected disasters are the norm, not the exception. Use the half-hour rule. Plan to leave a half hour earlier than you normally would in order to get there on time.
- Use disposable diapers or a diaper service.
- If it isn't dirty, don't clean it. Remember the 80/20 rule: 80% of the dirt is in 20% of the house. Clean the 20% area first. Leave the 80% for another time (like when the kids go to college).
- Learn to clean as you go. This makes less work at day's end.
- Keep one room in the house clean (like the living room) and muffins or cookies in the freezer or pantry for unexpected guests.
- Leave a list on the fridge of chores that need to be done. When visitors ask to help, have them choose a task.
- Have all visitors bring a special gift… Food!
- Screen all calls with an answering machine.
- Fill out government forms as soon as possible upon returning home.
- Order out for food or have a pizza night once a week.
- Use easily prepared foods. Frozen vegetables, premixed salad ingredients, pastas and sauces, BBQ chicken, etc.
- Collect time-saver recipes for meals in less than 20 minutes.
- Get showered, dressed and groomed every day. Avoid the bathrobed mother syndrome.
- Invest in a chest freezer or an extra fridge. Buy bulk supplies of all your most used grocery products (e.g., meat and bread).
- Make double batches of freezable meals (spaghetti sauces, casseroles, meatloaf, soups) and freeze for use on a hectic day.
- Learn to do two things at one time. (Vacuum the house or learn to cook dinner with baby in the front carrier.)
- Working mothers need to be especially good at time management. Make your regular chores part of baby's quality time.

YOUR HOME DOCTOR™ Mom

"NO-TIME" MANAGEMENT

Trade Secrets

- Quiet time is not a luxury but a necessity – to quench your soul.
- Pray, meditate or just sit and contemplate once a day.
- Learn to have realistic daily expectations.
- Learn to be ultra-organized and efficient.
- Simplify every aspect of your life.
- Don't view time as a container in which you have to place all the things that need to be done. View time as a candy bowl to pick and choose.
- Take one day at a time. It may seem impossible sometimes but try to enjoy every day and every development stage.
- Live in the present. We sometimes get too preoccupied waiting for the next stage that we don't enjoy the present one.
- Acknowledge your successes every day.
- Be kind to yourself. Remember that, believe it or not, you are only human. If you happen to forget, your kids will surely remind you when they are teenagers.
- Learn to relax. Let life wash over you like a warm summer shower, not a tidal wave.
- Remember, when your time management plan completely fails you, try to remain flexible and keep your sense of humor.
- Accept that there are some things in life you cannot change. Have the courage to change those things that you know you can.
- Learn when it is important to give your children your undivided attention. The concept of "No-Time" should never apply to your children.
- Educate yourself about being a mother and parent. This means reading books and magazines to learn. A good parenting magazine is often chock-full of helpful tips. Subscribe to one.
- Use the library. It is a treasure trove of information for both you and your children. They often have mother-tot groups and some even have babysitting.
- Use the Internet to find parenting and mother Net sites. Learn how to search for specific topics of interest.
- Talk to other mothers (including your own or your mother-in-law) to find out their trade secrets of motherhood.

Definitions

- **Stress** is physical, mental and emotional strain resulting from adapting to the changing demands of life and a feeling of loss of control of one's life. Stress can be from negative events as well as positive happenings like having a baby.

NUTRITION AND VITAMINS

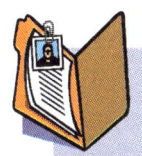

CASE STUDY

Henrietta was nine months postpartum when she was seen in the office.

"Can you recommend a good vitamin for me?" she asked. "I've been feeling so rundown lately."

During our discussion I discovered that Henrietta was trying to lose the weight that she had gained during her pregnancy. She was trying to do this by skipping breakfast and lunch each day. Unfortunately, by the time suppertime rolled around she was so ravenous that she had extra servings of dinner and continued to snack right up until she went to bed. Her snacks were generally high-fat, high-sugar "comfort foods" such as taco chips, ice cream and cookies because they were the snacks she craved the most. She was still getting up three times per night to breastfeed her infant and had recently restarted her menstrual periods.

I discussed nutritional needs and goals and how to achieve them. We also spent time reviewing weight loss strategies and essential vitamin and mineral requirements for breastfeeding moms.

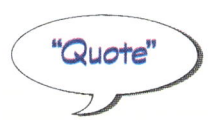

"Quote"

Become a nutritional commando. Search out and consume the snacks most valuable to your body. That's an order!

Eat well and so will your baby.

NUTRITION AND VITAMINS

TIPS

- The postpartum period is a perfect time to improve dietary habits especially if breastfeeding. Eat foods as close as possible to their natural state. The less processed the better.
- Make easy-to-prepare meals and snacks.
- Breastfeeding is a good time for you to relax and eat during the day, so grab a drink and snack each time you go to nurse the baby.
- Prepare prenatally by making freezer meals. Store them away for those days when cooking is too difficult.
- Ask friends and family to bring food instead of baby gifts!
- The average daily energy intake should be around 1200 kcal.
- A breastfeeding mother should increase her calorie consumption by 450 kcal/day.
- Women who breastfeed longer than six months should increase their energy intake an additional 200 kcal/day (to a total of 650 kcal extra per day).
- Nicotine (including secondhand smoke) should be avoided during breastfeeding, as it may increase baby's risk of respiratory tract problems and SIDS and decrease the milk supply.
- Naturopathic remedies, such as herbal teas and herbs, may affect nutrition and breastfeeding. Always check with your doctor before starting something like this.
- Vegetarian diets are often deficient in vitamins B12, D and calcium. Supplementation may be required.
- If you are breastfeeding, remember, you're still eating for two.
- Take care of yourself. This means eating regularly and not skipping meals or snacks. You will need the energy!
- Choose healthy nutritious foods. Try to eat small, nutritious meals every two to three hours (just like baby does) rather than three big meals per day.
- Eat to maintain your energy levels, promote healing, produce enough milk if breastfeeding and help in taking off extra pounds.
- Foods to choose: complex carbohydrates such as whole grain breads and cereals, legume's, wild rice and various fruits and vegetables.
- Limit your fat intake to less than 30% of your calories.
- Most women eat very well during pregnancy. Try to keep up with this same healthy eating after delivery.
- After your delivery and especially when breastfeeding, your body needs more calcium, folic acid, iron, magnesium, vitamins A, B6, C, D and zinc.
- Fat-soluble vitamins can build up and reach toxic levels if consumed in large doses. These include vitamins A, D, E and K.

NUTRITION AND VITAMINS
A DAILY CHART FOR BREASTFEEDING MOMS

GRAIN PRODUCTS
5 - 12 SERVINGS PER DAY

1 SERVING
Whole Wheat Bread . . . . .1 Slice
Cold Cereal 30g
Hot Cereal . . . . .175ml / 3/4 Cup

2 SERVINGS
Bran Muffin, Bagel or Bun 1
Rice or Pasta . . . . .250 ml / 1 Cup

☐ ☐ ☐ ☐ ☐ ☐ ☐ ☐ ☐ ☐

FRUITS AND VEGETABLES
5 - 10 SERVINGS PER DAY

1 SERVING
Raisins .60 ml / 42g
Medium Sized Fruit or Vegetable 1
Fresh/Frozen Fruit or Vegetables . . . . . 1/2 Cup
Salad . . . . .1 Cup
Juice . . . . .125 ml / 1/2 Cup

☐ ☐ ☐ ☐ ☐ ☐ ☐ ☐ ☐ ☐

MILK PRODUCTS
3 - 4 SERVINGS PER DAY

1 SERVING
Cheese 50g
Processed Cheese . . . . .50g / 2 Slices
Yogurt . . . . .175g / 3/4 Cup
Milk . . . . .250 ml / 1 Cup

1/2 SERVING
Cottage Cheese . . . . .250 ml / 1 Cup
Ice Cream . . . . .175 ml / 3/4 Cup
Pudding . . . . .125 ml / 1/2 Cup

☐ ☐ ☐

MEAT AND ALTERNATIVES
2 - 3 SERVINGS PER DAY

1 SERVING
Meat, Poultry or Fish . . . . .50 - 100g
Beans . . . . .125 - 250ml / 1/2 - 1 Cup
Peanut Butter . . . . .30ml / 2 tbsp
Canned Fish . . . . .50 - 100g / 1/3 - 2/3 Can
Tofu .100g / 1/3 Cup
Eggs . . . . .1 - 2

☐ ☐ ☐

Place a checkmark in the appropriate box each time you have a snack or meal.
It will help you make sure you get a balanced diet.
You may make photocopies of this page for continued daily use.

YOUR HOME DOCTOR™ Mom

NUTRITION AND VITAMINS

TIPS
Weight Loss Tips

- Take time losing the weight you gained during pregnancy. The slower the weight is lost, the more likely it will stay off.
- Diets rarely work. Behavior modification does. This means you need to change how, what and when you eat.
- Don't buy high-fat, high-calorie junk foods that you are likely to eat during those late night feedings. Avoid chips, cookies, ice cream, chocolate bars, candies, etc.
- Liquid diets, severely restricted diets and weight loss medications are not advisable.
- Eating small amounts regularly helps to promote weight loss.
- Weight loss of more than 1 kg per month (2 kg per month if overweight) is not advisable as it may result in:
  – An increase in maternal fatigue.
  – A decrease in milk supply.
- Your weight is a good guide of adequate nutrition. If your weight is dropping too quickly, your caloric intake is not high enough. The reverse is true if your weight stays high.

Fluid Tips

- The recommended fluid intake is six to eight glasses per day. Best choices are fruit juices, milk and water. The rule of thumb is to drink to quench your thirst (if your urine is dark yellow, you need to drink more; if your urine is light yellow or clear, you are drinking enough).
- You will need slightly more water if you had twins or triplets.
- Limit caffeine intake to a maximum of three cups per day. Caffeine can cause heart palpitations, anxiety and irritability and decreases the body's absorption of calcium.
- Caffeine is passed through the breastmilk and remains in your baby's body for many hours. Restrict your caffeine intake (e.g. coffee, tea, colas, chocolate, hot chocolate, iced tea) to one to two servings per day to avoid infant irritability and difficulty sleeping.
- Avoid alcohol when breastfeeding. It may affect the let down reflex. Alcohol can make the breastmilk taste bad for baby.
- Liquid supplements or nutrition drinks are an option if you find that you are skipping meals. These drinks usually contain a combination of vitamins, minerals, protein, fat and carbohydrates.

Vitamin and Mineral Tips

- It is always best to obtain vitamins and minerals from a well-balanced diet rather than through supplements.
- Always consult your doctor about the type and dose of vitamin supplements you are considering taking.

NUTRITION AND VITAMINS

TIPS
Vitamin and Mineral Tips

Calcium
- Getting enough calcium, especially if breastfeeding, is important. Otherwise you may lower your own bone density, placing you at increased risk of osteoporosis later in life.
- Mothers who do not drink milk must obtain calcium from other sources (e.g., yogurt, cheese, broccoli, spinach, almonds, sardines, canned salmon, tofu or through calcium supplements).

Folic Acid
- Should be taken when trying to get pregnant and after delivery.
- Found in foods such as liver, leafy greens and yeast products.

Iron (Needed to treat fatigue from anemia)
- Continue to take your prenatal vitamins, start iron supplements or increase red meats, beans, spinach or chick peas.
- Iron is best absorbed when taken with nondairy, calcium-rich foods (e.g., broccoli, almonds) or with foods containing vitamin C (citrus fruits, tomatoes).

Magnesium
- Found in nuts, milk products, wheat germ and cereal grains, green leafy vegetables, seafoods.

Vitamin A
- Found in milk products, green leafy or yellow fruits/vegetables.

Vitamin B6
- Found in pork, beef, fish, organ meats, seeds, whole grains.

Vitamin C (Important for healing)
- Some water-soluble vitamins including vitamin C are lost when cooked in water. Eat raw fruits and vegetables such as oranges, melons, broccoli, tomatoes, bell peppers.

Vitamin D
- Found in salmon, tuna, liver, egg yolk and fortified milks.

Other Essentials

Fiber (4 to 6 servings per day)
- Dietary fiber is crucial to get and keep your bowels moving. Sources include vegetables (brussels sprouts, cabbage, carrots, corn, green beans, lettuce); grains (brown rice, oatmeal, whole wheat or rye, unprocessed bran); fruits (apples, apricots, figs, oranges, pears, prunes, raisins); legume's (chick peas, kidney beans, lentils, soy beans).

Protein (2 to 3 servings per day)
- Protein is essential for healing and milk production. Choose lean meats, milk, tofu, legume's, eggs or cheese.

NUTRITION AND VITAMINS

Trade Secrets
What is transferred in breastmilk?

- One of the greatest concerns of breastfeeding mothers is what (if anything) will be passed through in the breast milk. The bottom line is, everything you eat or drink can be passed on in your breastmilk. So avoid the things you don't want baby exposed to.
- Some of the basic components of breastmilk remain unchanged by mother's diet. Breastmilk will consistently have enough of the minerals such as calcium, magnesium, phosphorus, sodium and potassium.
- Vigorous exercising and certain spices, vitamins and minerals, alcohol and caffeine often change the taste and content of breastmilk.
- Certain foods can give a strong taste to your breastmilk. The most common offenders are garlic, onions and cabbage.
- Don't automatically avoid fussy foods like cabbage, spices, chocolate or juices during breastfeeding unless it bothers you or your baby.
- Breastfed babies do not need to be given extra water during hot weather – just breastfeed more often. Breastmilk is 90% water!
- Babies labeled colicky may in fact have allergies or intolerances to certain foods. The most common food intolerance is milk, especially cow's milk. Other foods that occasionally cause trouble include egg whites, wheat, peanut butter, seafood, corn, citrus foods, tomatoes, strawberries and certain spices.
- Symptoms of intolerance include diarrhea, cramps, vomiting, bloating, eczema, irritability and a congested or runny nose.
- If you suspect an intolerance to a food, remove the food from your diet for at least seven days.
- It may take up to six hours for foods that you eat to change the taste of your breastmilk.
- Caffeine is a stimulant. Limit yourself to two cups per day.
- Avoid smoking and secondhand smoke.
- Avoid all recreational or street drugs, including alcohol.
- Avoid all medications, including prescription, over-the-counter, herbal, naturopathic, vitamins, etc., unless specifically approved of by your family doctor or pharmacist.
- You can continue to breastfeed your baby during a cold or "the flu." Your baby will not get your infection from the breastmilk. Wash your hands well before handling baby and drink plenty of fluids to replace the ones you are losing.
- Make sure that everyone involved in providing for your health knows that you are breastfeeding.
- Remember, you are what you eat, and so is your baby.

RELATIONSHIP CHANGES

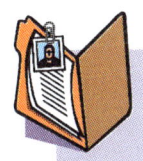

CASE STUDY

Carol came in to the office nine months after the birth of her son.

"My life is such a mess," she exclaimed. "My husband is upset that we never have any quality time together, my mother is upset that I never listen to her advice about raising the children, my friends are upset that I never call them anymore, my other children are upset that I am spending so much time with the baby, and my boss is upset that I haven't returned to work yet. Even the dog seems unhappy with me. The only person who isn't upset with me is the baby. I knew that things would change again with a new baby but I feel like I am living in relationship hell, with everyone wanting a piece of me... Help!"

Carol was discovering the magnitude of relationship changes after the birth of her third baby.

Our discussion outlined some of the major areas that Carol was having trouble with. I helped her devise a game plan to improve each of her high-priority relationships.

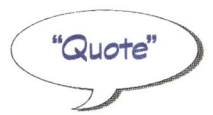

"Quote"

Flexibility is as important for relationship health as it is for physical health.

Communication is a two-way street.

Babies change things, especially relationships.

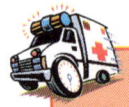

RELATIONSHIP CHANGES

WARNING
Go to your Doctor if you have ANY of the following:

- A feeling that you are losing control • Symptoms of depression
- Feeling isolated or negative
- Constant fighting or arguments with friends or family

GOALS
To better adapt to a major life change while maintaining important relationships.

TIPS

Your Partner
- Let's face it, your time together will decrease, but try to make it quality time. Make it part of an event in which you become more supportive of each other. Remember, parenting is a team sport.
- Your husband may not adapt to fatherhood as quickly as you do to motherhood. Give him gentle encouragement and time.
- The relationship with your partner, although the most important, is often the one that suffers the most after a new baby.
- Keep your partner involved in all decision making.

Your Parents
- Learn to rely on them for advice and babysitting.
- Keep them an active part of the excitement of your new baby.
- Try not to feel overwhelmed or negative about advice given.
- We all have different mothering styles. Don't feel guilty when you ignore unwanted advice from those you love. It's your baby.
- Remember, you will always be your parents' child.

Your Other Children
- Prepare them for the demands of the new baby by discussing how baby will affect their lives. Explain both the good and bad points, but concentrate on the good points.
- Continue to schedule special times for all your children.
- Actively include your children in the baby's care. They can be a great asset. Make a game out of all the work tasks.
- Major changes in your child's life, like toilet training, should be attempted early in your pregnancy or well after the new baby is born.
- Be prepared for sibling rivalry. Plan how you will deal with it.

Your Friends and Co-workers
- Make a point of contacting them at least once a month.
- Time for friendships will be in short supply. True friends (especially those with kids) will accept this and allow you appropriate down time to recover and adapt.
- Many of your interests will change. So may your friends.
- You will make many new friends, who are also parents.

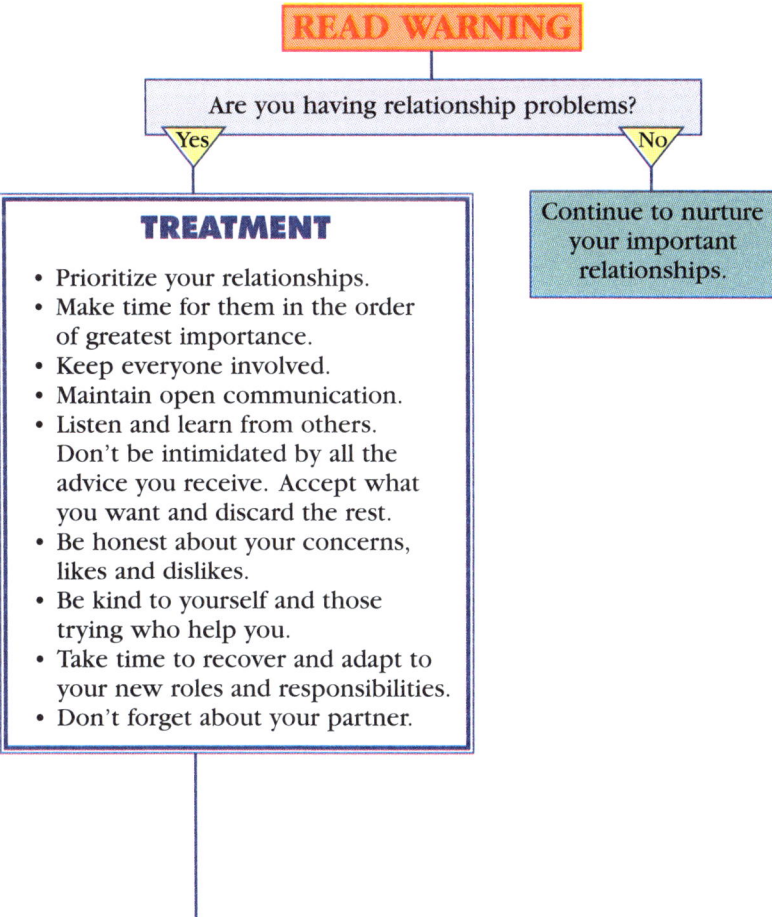

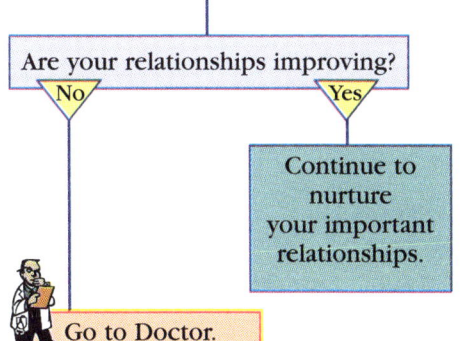

RELATIONSHIP CHANGES

READ WARNING

Are you having relationship problems?

Yes → **TREATMENT**

- Prioritize your relationships.
- Make time for them in the order of greatest importance.
- Keep everyone involved.
- Maintain open communication.
- Listen and learn from others. Don't be intimidated by all the advice you receive. Accept what you want and discard the rest.
- Be honest about your concerns, likes and dislikes.
- Be kind to yourself and those trying who help you.
- Take time to recover and adapt to your new roles and responsibilities.
- Don't forget about your partner.

No → Continue to nurture your important relationships.

Are your relationships improving?

Yes → Continue to nurture your important relationships.

No → Go to Doctor.

RELATIONSHIP CHANGES

Trade Secrets

- Having children can be very hard on relationships.
- Many couples experience an increase in conflict and a decrease in marriage satisfaction after their baby is born.
- Strategic plans for romance and conflict resolution are essential for relationship survival.
- Be kind to yourself, your partner, friends and family.
- Learn to deal with conflicts in a non-confrontational way.
- Flexibility and compromise are essential to maintain healthy relationships with those you care about.
- When arguments are heating up, cool down or go for a walk.
- Many problems arise from fatigue due to a lack of sleep. This is especially true in the first year of baby's life.
- Avoid criticism or sarcasm when dealing with others.
- The foundation of a happy relationship is best supported with communication. Invest in your relationships with time and effort and the dividends will be rich.
- Take five minutes at the beginning and end of each day to prepare for and catch up with your partner's daily events.
- Take time weekly to go out on a date with your partner. Even if it is only for a short walk, movie or a cup of coffee.
- Make time for yourself. When you short-change yourself you also short-change the ones you love.
- There are only 24 hours in the day. You will need to learn how to prioritize your time. Housework should suffer before any relationships do. Avoid the supermom syndrome!
- When out with your partner make a pact not to talk about the children for the first hour. Enjoy other topics of conversation with each other first.
- Make special time with your other children. Even reading books or playing a game while the baby naps or feeds is considered special time to a child.
- Be prepared: Becoming a mother may change the way you think about yourself.
- Learning how to balance the old you with the new you will help keep both of you happy.

Definitions

- **Relationship changes** are differences in how you deal with people, especially those closest to you.

SEX CONCERNS

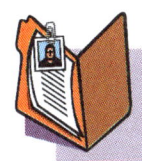

CASE STUDY (Normal Vaginal Birth)

Irene was seen in the office nine months after the birth of her first child.

"Doc, you have to help me get my sex drive back. Right now it doesn't even register on the libido meter. At first I thought it was just the new baby, the nighttime feedings and the general chaos of motherhood, but it's not getting any better. By the end of the day I'm so tired I have trouble staying awake through the evening news. In fact, by the time my head touches my pillow at night I'm already asleep. I used to be a very sexual person. I'm afraid motherhood is starting to make me celibate. My husband has been remarkably patient up until now, but I know he is starting to get a little frustrated too."

Irene was having difficulty with her sexual health, especially balancing the demands of motherhood with her sexuality.

Our ensuing discussion uncovered a combination of sleep deprivation, increased work demands and a general reduction in the time Irene and her husband were able to spend together as a couple. It was time to get back to the basics by concentrating on treating the cause of the problems, not the symptoms.

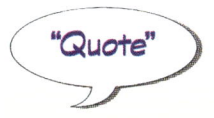

"Quote"

Kids in your bed at night provide an effective means of birth control and a healthy dose of sexual repression.

Good conversation is the world's best aphrodisiac.

A good lubricant is a poor substitute for proper arousal.

SEX CONCERNS

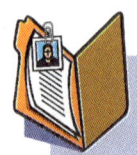

CASE STUDY (Traumatic Vaginal Birth)

Nicole was seen in the office two months after delivery.

"I expected my husband and I would be having sex again by now, but after the forceps delivery, the episiotomy, the fourth-degree tear and all those stitches, I'm terrified of him coming anywhere near me," she lamented. "I'm still finding it hard to sit down to have a bowel movement, and the incision still sometimes aches and burns. Is this normal? How long before I get back to normal?"

Examination revealed a tender ridge of scar tissue along the incision site of the episiotomy and a healing fourth degree tear. The anus was working normally. There was no evidence of infection.

Nicole was having trouble returning to regular sexual activity after her very traumatic birth experience.

We discussed the expected course of healing following a traumatic birth such as hers and the various options for sexual intimacy that did not include sexual intercourse.

Nicole healed gradually and returned to full sexual relations, including intercourse, about six months after her delivery.

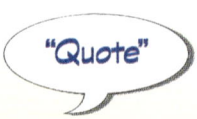

"Quote"

Traumatic births can lead to traumatic sex. Ample time to heal, a good lubricant and your partner's patience will usually return you to normal sexual relations.

There is more to intimacy than intercourse.

SEX CONCERNS

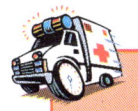

WARNING

Go to your Doctor if you have ANY of the following:

- Pain with intercourse • A sudden increase in vaginal bleeding
- Fever above 38.5°C (101.3°F) • Vaginal discharge
- Involuntary vaginal muscle contractions

GOALS

To return to a mutually satisfying sexual relationship.

TIPS

- People require time to adjust to their new role as parents. Infant demands and altered sleep patterns combined with physical changes can lead to physical exhaustion and a decreased desire for sexual intimacy.
- You may experience feelings of sexual inadequacy due to changes in your physical appearance. Stretch marks, excess weight, change in breast size and excess skin may make you feel less desirable. Communicating with your partner is vital during this period for reassurance, acceptance and support.
- Intercourse can sometimes be restarted two weeks after a normal delivery. (Exceptions: traumatic births and C–sections.)
- Sexual expression and intimacy can be accomplished by means other than sexual intercourse. Try caressing, mutual masturbation, oral sex, massage or other forms of stimulation.
- Women sometimes avoid intercourse after delivery because they fear pregnancy, pain or due to concerns that she is changed.
- Pregnancy within the first two to four weeks after delivery is rare but not impossible. (See Birth Control page 25).
- Intercourse may be uncomfortable for the first few months after delivery because of changes in the vaginal tissue.
- Breastfeeding women may experience vaginal dryness. Try a lubricating jelly to increase comfort.
- Couples with the most active sex lives often schedule sex into their busy lives. Sex doesn't have to be spontaneous to be great.
- To protect your passion, keep a sense of humor, the lines of communication open and a lock on the bedroom door.
- Forget what it was like before kids. Things have changed, adapt.
- Find reliable babysitters as soon as possible. They are an absolute necessity. Never cancel a babysitter or return home early. Enjoy your special time together.
- Make your bedroom into a love sanctuary, not a nursery.
- After vaginal delivery you may find your vagina a little larger and sex a little less satisfying. Remember to do your Kegel exercises.

SEX CONCERNS

TIPS (Continued)

- Be spontaneous. If an opportunity presents itself, close the bedroom door and take advantage of a few moments together.
- Try the six-second kiss. Holding your kisses longer re-ignites the flame. It also gives you something to anticipate later.
- Breastfeeding women sometimes experience breastmilk leakage during orgasm. Some couples find this unacceptable. Apply pressure to the breasts, place towels underneath or feed baby prior to lovemaking to prevent this.
- Some women have sensual feelings during breastfeeding. You should not become alarmed by this experience. This pleasure is natural and occurs because of the release of the hormone oxytocin. This should in no way be confused with a sexually inappropriate act.
- Societal pressures influence women and men, to believe that breasts are for sexual pleasure. Often women choose not to breastfeed because of the emotional turmoil caused by societal pressure. Parents should discuss their beliefs about breasts with each other before ruling out breastfeeding as a feeding option.
- Some research suggests that the use of a family bed, where parents and their children share the same bed, may promote closeness and bonding. Couples should discuss issues such as these before having children to better decide what is best for their family. Children sleeping in your bed can be a strain on your sex life.
- Women often find it more comfortable to be on top during intercourse, especially during the first few months postpartum. This position allows the woman to better control the amount and depth of penile thrusting.
- The missionary position may be uncomfortable after having a baby due to full, tender lactating breasts. This may be especially true after a cesarean section birth, episiotomy or a traumatic birth.
- Experiment with various positions and ways of making love. Find positions that are comfortable and allow you to control the rate and speed of penetration. Kneeling on top or the "cupped spoon" position are two of the best to start with.
- Learn to find romance and passion in everyday occurrences.
- Use the VCR to your advantage. Put in a movie for the kids, close the door and do what comes naturally.
- Wake early to have sex, rather than waiting to the end of the day.
- Great sex is a learned skill. It takes good communication and plenty of practice.
- Make a sex "wish list" and ask for what you would like.

SEX CONCERNS

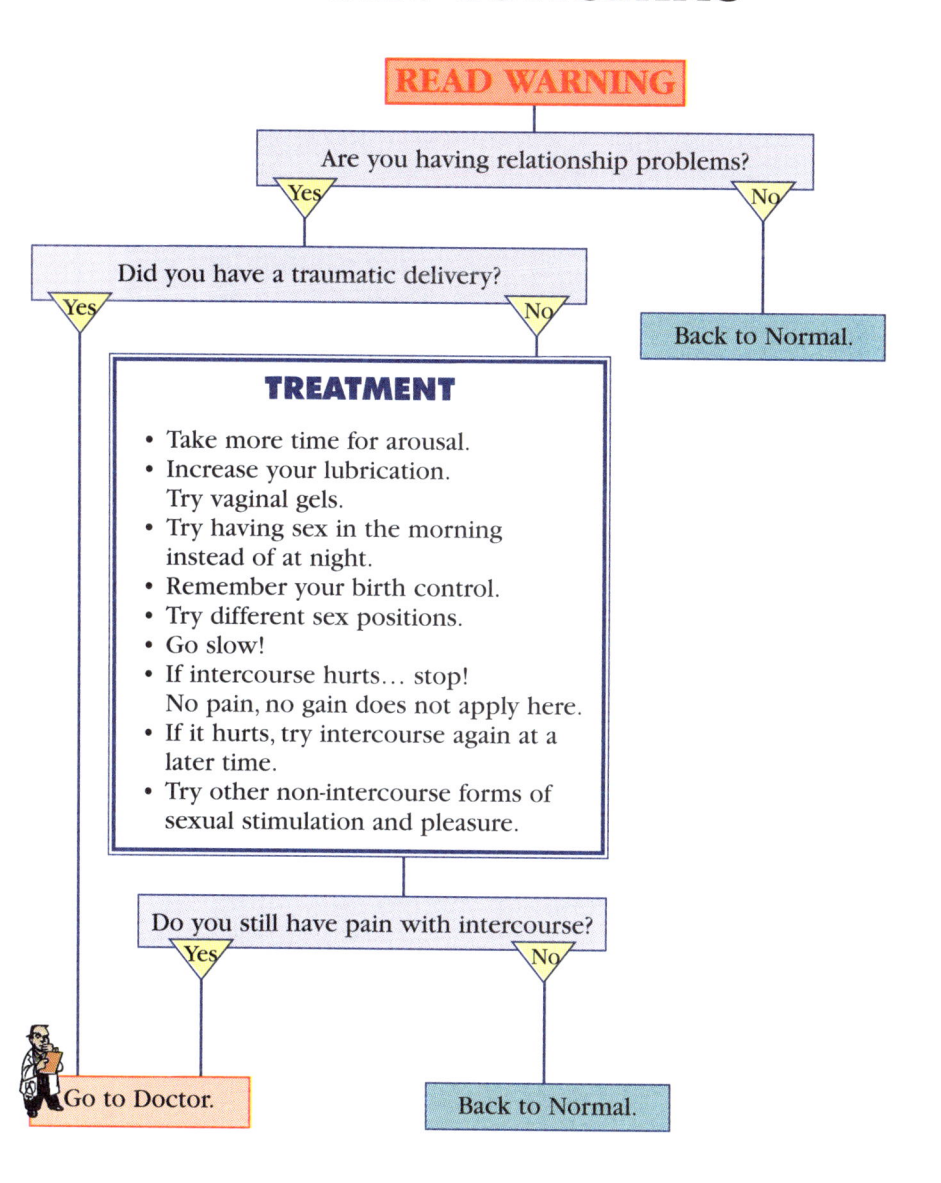

READ WARNING

Are you having relationship problems?

- Yes → Did you have a traumatic delivery?
  - Yes → Go to Doctor.
  - No → TREATMENT
- No → Back to Normal.

TREATMENT

- Take more time for arousal.
- Increase your lubrication. Try vaginal gels.
- Try having sex in the morning instead of at night.
- Remember your birth control.
- Try different sex positions.
- Go slow!
- If intercourse hurts… stop! No pain, no gain does not apply here.
- If it hurts, try intercourse again at a later time.
- Try other non-intercourse forms of sexual stimulation and pleasure.

Do you still have pain with intercourse?

- Yes → Go to Doctor.
- No → Back to Normal.

SEX CONCERNS

Trade Secrets

- People always require time to recover and adjust to their new role as parents, regardless of the number of children.
- Open, honest communication and slow, sensual sex is the key.
- Having kids can be hard on your relationship. Many couples experience an increase in conflict and a decrease in marriage satisfaction after the baby is born. Strategic plans for romance and conflict resolution are essential for marital survival.
- Be nice to each other and sex will soon follow.
- Be realistic. Having children changes your sex life. How good it gets depends on how committed and imaginative you can be.
- The sleepless nights and demands of motherhood will eventually get better. Know that things do improve and heal with time.
- Remember, good, candid conversation is the best foreplay.
- Do not abuse drugs or fake orgasms, both can lead to problems.
- Many women have difficulty achieving orgasm with vaginal intercourse and need direct clitoral stimulation for orgasm.
- An orgasm is an orgasm regardless of the cause. Try different forms of stimulation to obtain the desired effect.
- Remember to pleasure each other in nonsexual ways too.
- Your return to sex will depend upon the nature of your delivery.

Definitions

- **Dyspareunia** is painful intercourse.
- **Episiotomy** is an incision, made by the doctor, of the external female genital organs in order to assist in the delivery of a baby.
- **Fourth-degree tear** is a vaginal tear extending into the rectum.
- **Masturbation** is the stimulation of one's own genitals.
- **Orgasm** is the pinnacle of sexual excitement.
- **Sexuality** is the sexual expressiveness of an individual.

Synonyms

- Coitus • Intercourse • Fornication • Masturbation • Oral sex
- Penis-vagina intercourse • Sexual intercourse • Vaginal sex

Medications/Treatments

- **Lubricants** may help reduce vaginal dryness, irritation and chafing during intercourse.
- **Sex toys** (vibrators, etc.) heighten or expand sexual experiences.

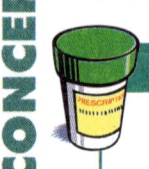

SKIN PROBLEMS

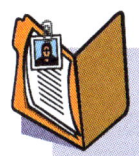

CASE STUDY

Katrina was nine months postpartum when she came in to the office.

"Isn't there anything that I can do for these stretch marks?" she asked. "I must have tried every product on the market by now and none of them seem to have done a thing. Between the oils, creams, vitamin E, massages, herbal therapies, mud treatments, etc., I must have spent close to $500. What does the medical profession have to offer?"

On examination Katrina had extensive stretch marks on her thighs, breasts and abdomen.

We discussed the cause of stretch marks and the lack of any reliable and proven treatment. She was, however, pleased with the knowledge that the redness of her stretch marks would fade and the stretch marks would naturally heal over the next year or two.

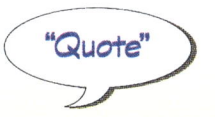

"Quote"

Aromatic oil massages and therapeutic body rubs don't stop stretch marks... they cause pregnancies.

God grant me the serenity to accept the things I cannot change, the courage to change the things I can, and the wisdom to know the difference.

— Anonymous

SKIN PROBLEMS

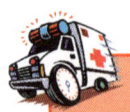

WARNING
Go to your Doctor if you have ANY of the following:

- Skin rashes • Skin eruptions • Itchiness
- Yellow coloring of skin, dark urine or pale stools • Hives
- Sudden swelling of the hands, feet or face
- Difficulty breathing or swallowing

SYMPTOMS

- Changes in skin texture, appearance and color are common in pregnancy and in the postpartum period.

GOALS

To ease the discomfort of skin conditions.

TIPS

Acne
- Do not use any acne treatments until you first check with your doctor. This is especially important when breastfeeding.
- Gently clean your skin twice daily with mild soap and water.
- Avoid all exfoliants, brushes, pads, face creams, foundations, facials, face scrubs and harsh cleansers. Avoid picking and squeezing your pimples.
- Use oil-free make up and sunscreens (SPF 15 or higher).

Black and Bloodshot Eyes (broken blood vessels)
- Usually result from pushing hard during childbirth.
- Apply warm compresses. These will resolve within three weeks.

Chapped Hands and Dry Skin
- Use a moisturizer. The more thick and greasy the better. Choose moisturizers without perfumes or preservatives.
- Always moisturize your hands after they have been in water.
- Avoid excessively hot baths and showers, bubble baths, body washes and soaps (except for soaping hands, groin and armpits). Soaps tend to dry the skin and remove natural protective oils.
- Wear vinyl gloves with cotton liners when cleaning.
- Apply petroleum jelly at night to soften and heal chapped hands.
- Dry skin does not cause wrinkles. Sun exposure does.
- Use a vaporizer in your house to increase the humidity.
- Avoid using harsh cleaners, chemicals and detergents.

Darkening of Skin on Face (Melasma)
- This often fades after the birth of your baby.
- Certain creams (e.g., Retin–A, Viquin Forte) may help to resolve melasma. They cannot be used in breastfeeding women.
- Sun exposure worsens this condition. Avoid suntanning. Always use a sunscreen with an SPF factor of 15 or greater.

SKIN PROBLEMS

TIPS

Darkening of Moles and Freckles
- This is normal. The color may lighten after birth.
- A changing skin lesion must always be checked by a doctor.

Darkening of Skin, Nipples and Areola
- This is due to hormonal changes. The colour may lighten after birth.

Excessive Hair Growth
- Try shaving, waxing or tweezers to remove unwanted hairs.
- Check with your doctor before using bleaches and depilatories.
- The only permanent method of hair removal is electrolysis.
- All sudden increase in hair growth must be checked by a doctor.

Greasy skin
- Keep your skin clean. Use a mild hypoallergenic soap such as Dove, Allenbury's, Neutrogena and bare hands to wash.
- Avoid moisturizers, astringents, toners, etc.

Hair loss
- Very common after childbirth. It is usually most severe approximately four months after delivery.
- Normal hair loss slows during pregnancy. Your body catches up with normal hair growth while pushing out the old hairs.
- Don't worry, it will stop long before you go bald. The thickness of hair usually returns to normal within six months.
- There are no special diet, vitamin, health food or over-the-counter products useful for hair loss.
- Try keeping your hair shade slightly darker and have a perm every three months to give your hair more body.

Skin Tags
- A floppy growth of skin found in high-friction areas, often under the breast, armpits or along the neckline.
- Sometimes these shrink after birth. Often they need to be surgically removed. See your doctor about treatment.

Stretch Marks
- Start as pink/purple lines found mostly on breasts, abdomen, thighs and buttocks. They slowly fade to silver streaks.
- Stretch marks are not preventable as stretching occurs beneath the skin surface. This is why skin creams will not erase them.
- Don't waste your money on creams, pills or laser treatments.

Sweating and Hot Flashes
- Very common, especially in the first few days after delivery.
- This is the way the body rids extra fluids after delivery. They may be associated with chills but there should be no fever.
- Increase your fluid intake and take your temperature.
- Avoid alcohol and caffeine. Wear cotton clothing.

YOUR HOME DOCTOR™ Mom

SKIN PROBLEMS

Trade Secrets

- Many of the skin changes that occur during pregnancy will fade or disappear shortly after delivery.
- About 90% of women will get stretch marks. There are no good treatments. Fortunately, they fade over one to two years. No creams, vitamins, diets, minerals, health foods, naturopathic, holistic or over-the-counter remedies have been shown to work. Save your money and don't get duped by 1–800–RIP–OFFS or mail order remedies for this natural and self healing condition.
- Most women experience some changes in skin appearance before or after delivery. Most are natural and common responses to normal hormonal changes.
- Acne is a hereditary condition. It is an oil problem within the skin and not on the skin. It has little to do with cleanliness.
- Be especially careful of any product you use while you are pregnant, trying to get pregnant or breastfeeding.
- See your family doctor or dermatologist if your skin condition is worsening or causing you concern despite treatment.

Definitions

- **Areola** is the circular area surrounding the nipple.
- **Linea Nigra** is a pigmented brown line on the anterior abdominal wall running between the belly button and the pelvic bone.
- **Skin Eruptions** are visible lesions on the skin.

Synonyms

- Acne: pimples, zits, blemishes, comedones, whiteheads, blackheads, papules, cysts, pustules
- Chapped hands or dry skin: eczema, dermatitis
- Excessive hair growth: hirsutism, hypertrichosis
- Hair loss: balding, thinning

Medications/Treatments

- **Antibiotics** are used to treat bacterial skin infections.
- **Baking soda baths** relieve itchy skin conditions.
- **Cortisone creams/ointments** are used to reduce skin swelling, inflammation, eczema and itch.
- **Cryotherapy** uses liquid nitrogen to burn off benign skin lesions.
- **Moisturizing creams** and lotions (e.g., Alpha Keri, Moisturel, Nutraderm) seal moisture into the skin.

URINARY PROBLEMS

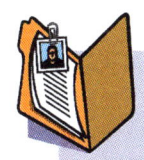

CASE STUDY

Juanita was two weeks postpartum when she came in to the office.

"I realize it is normal to be going to the bathroom a lot for the first few days after a baby is born, but this is ridiculous," she lamented. "I am going to the bathroom every half hour whether I want to or not. Most of the time I am only getting a little dribble out. Since yesterday I have noticed that it hurts when I pee, and I don't think it is from my episiotomy stitches."

Juanita was slightly flushed with a temperature of 38.5°C (101.3°F). She had some slight discomfort just above her pubic bone (the bladder) but not when pressing over her kidneys. She had no vaginal bleeding or lochia. Her urine tested positive for blood and pus cells, confirming a urinary tract infection.

Juanita had developed a postpartum urinary tract infection.

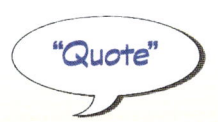

"Quote"

Urinary tract infections in the postpartum period are like Ninja. They strike suddenly and without warning under the cover of darkness.

URINARY PROBLEMS

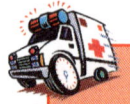

WARNING
Go to your Doctor if you have ANY of the following:

- Fever above 38.5°C (101.3°F) • Difficult or painful urination • Chills
- Dizziness • Fainting spells • Pelvic/groin pain
- Vaginal bleeding or discharge • Blood in your urine
- Constant or one-sided backache • Nausea and vomiting.

SYMPTOMS

- Urge to urinate (pee) frequently • Passing only small amounts
- Burning or discomfort when urinating • Lower abdominal discomfort
- Getting up at night to pee • Having to go urgently • Blood or pus in the urine

GOALS
To cure the infection, prevent spread of infection to the kidney and prevent recurring infections.

TIPS

- Many women experience some difficulty urinating the first few hours to days after childbirth.
- Make sure you urinate within six hours of delivery.
- Drink plenty of water or other noncaffeinated fluids. This means at least six to eight glasses per day.
- Cranberry juice is helpful for treating bladder infections.
- Do not hold your urine: go to the bathroom when you feel the urge. "Holding it" can increase the chances of infection.
- Empty your bladder completely each time. Leaning forward while urinating may help squeeze the bladder empty.
- Try straddling the toilet when urinating to prevent the stinging of urine touching sensitive episiotomy repairs.
- Avoid using perfumed perineal sprays, soaps, panty liners or vaginal deodorants, bubble baths, bath oils and douches.
- Use white toilet paper only. Always wipe from front to back.
- Wear breathable, non-constricting underwear (cotton is best).
- Get urine checked at the first sign of a urinary tract infection.
- Use a warm water bottle or heating pad for the relief of abdominal discomfort or sit in a warm sitz bath.
- When still bleeding in the postpartum period, cleanse the perineal area frequently with a squirt bottle (peribottle) filled with warm water and a capful of mineral oil. Remember to spray from front to back.
- Change tampons and pads frequently.
- Empty your bladder before and after sexual intercourse.

URINARY PROBLEMS

READ WARNING

Do you have any of the following when urinating?
- Going frequently and/or only small amounts.
- Burning sensation and/or blood.
- Lower abdominal pain.
- Waking at night to urinate (more than usual).
- Having to go urgently (you can't hold your urine)

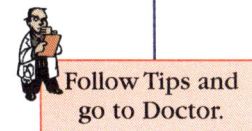

Yes → Follow Tips and go to Doctor.

No ↓

PREVENTIVE TREATMENT

- Drink plenty of fluids (water and fruit juices, including cranberry juice, are the best).
- Reduce coffee, tea, alcohol and cola drinks.
- Don't hold your urine. When you have to go… Go!
- Urinate before and after sexual intercourse (sex).
- Wear cotton underwear and loose-fitting clothing.
- Always wipe the vagina from front to back after urinating.
- Keep the vagina and anus very clean.
- Change pads and tampons frequently.

Go to your Doctor if you suspect that you may be developing a bladder infection.

YOUR HOME DOCTOR™ Mom

URINARY PROBLEMS

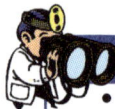

Trade Secrets

- Frequent urination after delivery and the numbness of the urethra from labor and delivery sometimes make it difficult to detect a bladder infection. Frequent testing is the secret.
- The bladder may be bruised, squashed, or paralyzed after childbirth. This along with medications and excess fluid loss during delivery may lead to difficulty getting the bladder back to work for a while.
- Bladder sensation is often reduced after delivery. Try to urinate every four hours after delivery.
- Kidney infections occur from spread of bacteria from the bladder. This is another good reason to urinate every two to three hours.
- Bladder infections are common after urinary catheter use.
- Yeast infections are common after antibiotic treatment.
- Incontinence is usually due to weak pelvic floor muscles. (See page 79 for exercises that can help).

Definitions

- **Antibiotics** are medicines used to treat specific infections.
- **Dysuria** is pain when urinating.
- **Frequency** is having to urinate often.
- **Lochia** is the fluid that comes from the vagina after childbirth.
- **Nocturia** is having to get up at night to urinate.
- **Perineal** refers to the area around the vagina.
- **Sexual intercourse** is "having sex," copulating or fornicating.
- **Urination** is passing water. Also known as voiding or peeing.
- **Urinary tract infection** is a bacterial infection of the bladder.

Synonyms

- Cystitis • Not pyelonephritis (this is a kidney infection)
- Urinary Tract Infection • UTI

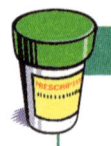

Medications/Treatments

- **Acetaminophen** is used to treat pain and fever.
- **Antibiotics** are prescribed to treat infections. Do NOT self-medicate. Finish all your prescribed antibiotics.
- **Bladder anesthetic pills** (pyridium) can help reduce discomfort.
- **A bladder catheter** is a tube placed in your bladder to help you empty it. This is normally done if you cannot urinate within six to eight hours after delivery.
- **Cranberry juice** is used to help treat urinary infections. It helps to reduce the growth of bacteria in the bladder.
- **Urine analysis** and urine culture are used to diagnose infections.

VAGINAL BLEEDING/DISCHARGE

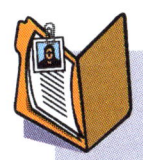

CASE STUDY

Anna attended her doctor's appointment at four weeks postpartum to discuss a number of her concerns.

"At first," she stated, "my bleeding seemed to be slowing down, but this past week I started bleeding heavier again. It also has a bad smell to it. Just yesterday I started getting a fever and chills. What do you think is wrong? This didn't happen after my first daughter was born."

Anna had a temperature of 38.5°C (101.3°F) and her uterus was very tender on palpation.

A diagnosis of endometritis (infection of the uterus lining) was made and she was started on antibiotics. An ultrasound of the uterus was also arranged to rule out any retained placental fragments, which might have required removal by surgery.

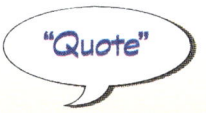

"Quote"

The larger the blood clots, the heavier the blood flow.

Gradual slowing of vaginal bleeding is another sign the uterus is returning to its pre-pregnancy state (from a pumpkin back to a plum) – an evolution that (amazingly) takes only two to six weeks.

YOUR HOME DOCTOR™ Mom

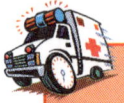

VAGINAL BLEEDING/DISCHARGE

WARNING
Go to your Doctor if you have ANY of the following:

- Fever above 38.5°C (101.3°F) • Clots larger than half your palm
- Increasing or continuous abdominal pain • Pad changes are required more frequently than every two hours • Dizziness or faintness
- Increasing fatigue • Shortness of breath • Chest pain
- Heart rate greater than 100 beats per minute • Lochia has foul odor

SYMPTOMS

- Postpartum vaginal bleeding is initially bright red then changes to pink and then to whitish-yellow. Initially the rate of flow is similar to a period but may contain clots or fragments of tissue. The flow normally slows, then stops in three to six weeks.

GOALS

To discover the cause of vaginal bleeding and lochia production and then determine whether treatment is required.

TIPS

- Bleeding or lochia after delivery usually slowly tapers off over two to six weeks. It may initially be as heavy as a normal period.
- Use sanitary napkins (maxipads) not tampons after delivery and for at least the first six weeks. Change pads frequently and keep track of the number of pads used each day.
- Massage the lower abdomen to help your uterus contract.
- Breastfeeding helps the uterus contract more quickly.
- Increased bleeding, especially after the first week, usually means you are doing too much, too soon.
- It is normal to feel a small gush of bleeding with increased activity or when getting out of bed. The bleeding should quickly stop with rest (this means lying down).
- Both baths or showers are okay during this time.
- Watch for any signs of infection: fevers, chills, a sudden onset of tiredness, lochia odor, lower abdominal pain, increased blood flow, passing large clots or feeling flushed.
- Keep your fluid intake up. The more you bleed, the more noncaffeinated fluids you need to drink. Rule of thumb: each time you change a pad have a large glass of water or juice.
- Use a peribottle (filled with warm water and a capful of mineral/baby oil) to rinse clean each time you use the toilet and before you apply a fresh pad.
- Some women find using their maternity underwear more comfortable for the first few weeks and when wearing pads.

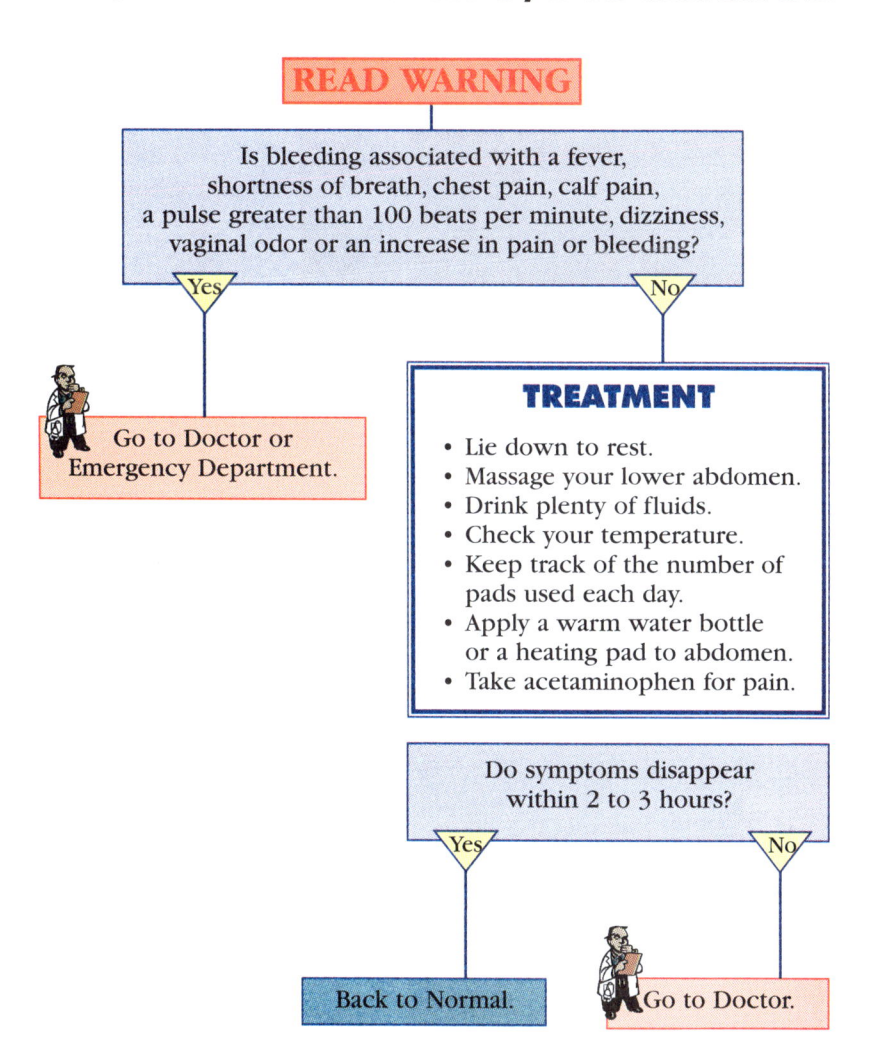

VAGINAL BLEEDING/DISCHARGE

READ WARNING

Is bleeding associated with a fever, shortness of breath, chest pain, calf pain, a pulse greater than 100 beats per minute, dizziness, vaginal odor or an increase in pain or bleeding?

Yes: Go to Doctor or Emergency Department.

No:

TREATMENT

- Lie down to rest.
- Massage your lower abdomen.
- Drink plenty of fluids.
- Check your temperature.
- Keep track of the number of pads used each day.
- Apply a warm water bottle or a heating pad to abdomen.
- Take acetaminophen for pain.

Do symptoms disappear within 2 to 3 hours?

Yes: Back to Normal.

No: Go to Doctor.

VAGINAL BLEEDING/DISCHARGE

Trade Secrets

- Higher risks of abnormal postpartum bleeding occur with: multiple pregnancies (e.g., twins), very fast or very slow labors, large infants, forceps use, retained placental fragments or infection, a previous postpartum bleed or a maternal bleeding problem.
- Lochia color usually starts bright red and changes to a brown discharge over six weeks. Brown discharge is older blood and is not abnormal unless you have other warning signs.
- Lochia is composed of the tissue, blood, mucus and debris left in the uterus after delivery. It is usually heaviest the first week after delivery.
- The amount of vaginal bleeding often has a direct correlation with the number of children you have at home, and therefore the more difficult it is to slow down and rest.

Definitions

- **Antibiotics** are medicines used to treat specific infections.
- **Endometritis** is an infection in the lining of the uterus.
- **Forceps** are metal clasp devices used to assist in delivery.
- **Hemorrhage** means bleeding.
- **Lochia** is the discharge from the vagina after delivery.
- **Postpartum hemorrhage** is the loss of one or more pints of blood during or after the passage of the placenta.
- **Palpation** is gentle pressure with the hand.
- **Retained placental fragments** are pieces of afterbirth left in the uterus after the delivery of the baby and placenta.
- **Vacuum extraction** is the use of a vacuum device to assist in delivery.

Synonyms

- Postpartum bleeding • Postpartum flow • Postpartum hemorrhage
- Vaginal discharge • Vaginal flow

Medications/Treatments

- **Acetaminophen** is used to treat pain and fever.
- **Antibiotics** are prescribed to treat uterine infections. DO NOT self–medicate with leftover or someone else's antibiotics. Always finish your antibiotics as prescribed.
- **Blood transfusions** are sometimes needed for heavy bleeding.
- **D&C** (dilation and curettage) is surgery sometimes needed to clean out the leftover pieces of placenta that cause bleeding.
- **IV therapy** is used to replace mild or moderate blood loss.
- **Oxytocin, ergotomine** or **prostaglandins** promote the contraction of the uterus and thereby reduce vaginal flow.

VARICOSE VEINS

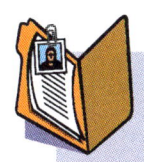

CASE STUDY

Betty came in to the office fourteen weeks after the birth of her second baby.

"I'm here to get something done about my legs," she exclaimed. "These varicose veins have been causing me grief the whole pregnancy. Even now they ache if I stand too long. I certainly don't want to end up with legs like my mother had. Her varicose veins were just awful and she suffered terribly. I thought maybe we should start a little proactive treatment program for my legs now before it gets too late."

Examination of Betty's legs showed some fairly significant varicose veins. They had definitely worsened during her last pregnancy despite her wearing support hose throughout the pregnancy and beyond. Unfortunately, Betty had a very strong family history of varicose veins that was working against her good efforts. She had no other medical problems and her examination was otherwise normal.

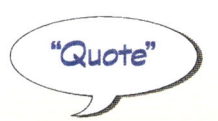

"Quote"

Varicose veins are a progressive problem.
They always get worse over time.
Much like the subject matter on the
Jerry Springer show.

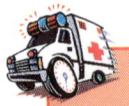

VARICOSE VEINS

> **WARNING**
> ***Go to your Doctor if you have ANY of the following:***
> - Legs or veins are red, hot, swollen or tender to touch (phlebitis)
> - Trouble walking • Excessive leg pain or cramps
> - Changing skin color or skin ulcer develops on legs
> - Shooting pains in the leg

SYMPTOMS

- Blue, purple or red bulging lines under the skin in the legs. They may be painless or cause symptoms such as heaviness, aching, swelling, burning, restlessness and tiredness. Varicose veins can also develop and cause symptoms in the vulva.

GOALS

To improve symptoms or cosmetic appearance.

TIPS

- Varicose veins are blue, bumpy, swollen and stretched veins usually in the legs.
- Spider veins are a type of varicose veins. They are very fine, like a spider web. They can develop anywhere and often are present in those with regular varicose veins.
- If varicose veins run in your family start preventive treatment.
- Treatment includes Exercise, Elevation and Support. Exercising leg and foot muscles helps pump blood and fluids out of the legs. Start walking daily – take your baby for a stroll. Elevating the legs helps to "drain the veins." Support stockings work as a pump to help remove extra fluid, reducing swelling and relieving discomfort.
- Wear proper varicose vein compression panty hose or thigh-highs. As a second choice use support panty hose with greater than 20% lycra. Put your stockings on before you get out of bed in the morning.
- Reduce weight and avoid long periods of standing or sitting.
- Avoid wearing tight clothing (belts, pants, girdles, knee-highs, etc.).
- Wear lace up shoes if you have swelling in your feet.
- Have your veins checked by a vein specialist after the baby is delivered. You don't have to wait until you have had all your children before you do something about your varicose veins.
- Regular treatment of veins between children helps in their control. The smaller the veins, the more successful the treatment.
- Elevating the foot of your bed improves nighttime blood flow.
- Eat healthy, nutritious meals. Reduce salt and increase vitamin C.
- Stop smoking and avoid secondhand smoke.

VARICOSE VEINS

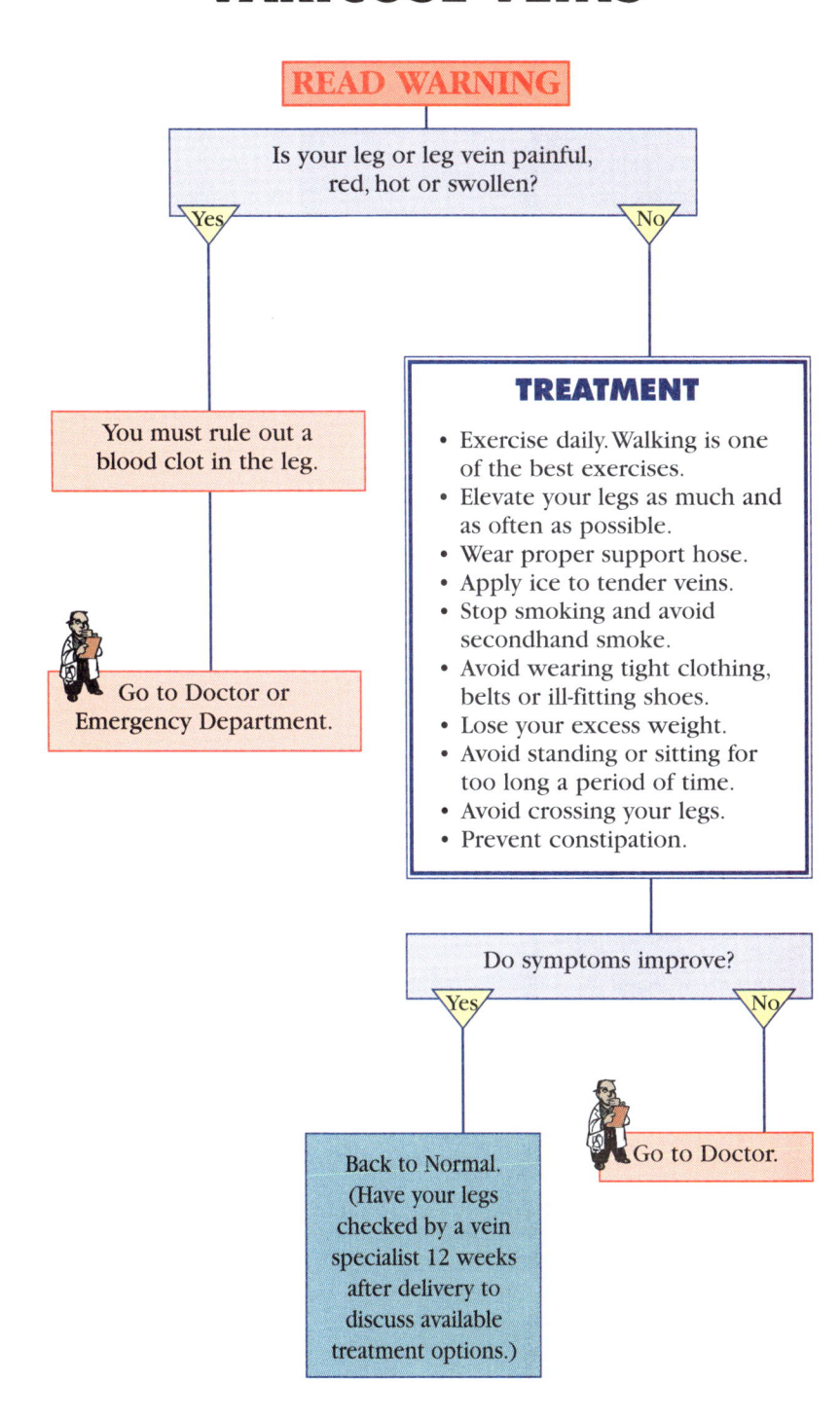

READ WARNING

Is your leg or leg vein painful, red, hot or swollen?

Yes → You must rule out a blood clot in the leg. Go to Doctor or Emergency Department.

No →

TREATMENT

- Exercise daily. Walking is one of the best exercises.
- Elevate your legs as much and as often as possible.
- Wear proper support hose.
- Apply ice to tender veins.
- Stop smoking and avoid secondhand smoke.
- Avoid wearing tight clothing, belts or ill-fitting shoes.
- Lose your excess weight.
- Avoid standing or sitting for too long a period of time.
- Avoid crossing your legs.
- Prevent constipation.

Do symptoms improve?

Yes → Back to Normal. (Have your legs checked by a vein specialist 12 weeks after delivery to discuss available treatment options.)

No → Go to Doctor.

VARICOSE VEINS

Trade Secrets

- Varicose veins may be minimized, by reducing the extra pressure on the veins in the legs.
- It's estimated that up to 40% of all pregnant women develop varicose veins. Many will partially resolve after delivery.
- Exercises like walking and cycling help improve varicose veins.
- Varicose veins are a progressive disease. Varicose veins always get worse with time. Early treatment makes good sense.
- Varicose veins have an increased risk of phlebitis (inflammation) or blood clot formation (thrombosis) with a possibility of clot transfer to the lungs (pulmonary embolus).
- Treatment controls but does not prevent varicose veins.
- Causes include genetics, pregnancy (hormones, increased blood volume, slowed circulation, and weight of uterus blocking pelvic veins), and prolonged standing or sitting.

Definitions

- **Phlebitis** is inflammation of a vein.
- **Thrombosis** is the blockage of a blood vessel.
- **Thrombophlebitis** is inflammation and blockage of a vein.
- **Vulva** is the outside folds (lips) that protect the vagina and the clitoris.

Synonyms

- Spider Veins • Telangectasia • Varicosities • Venous Changes

Medications/Treatments

- **Anti-inflammatories** or aspirin may help with discomfort. Do not use if breastfeeding. Do not use these regularly.
- **Compressive therapy** with fitted support stockings is highly recommended. These stockings promote improved blood flow from the feet up by graduated sock pressures gradients.
- **Exercise** after delivery assists circulation by strengthening the leg muscles. These muscles are the pumps that remove fluid and swelling from your legs.
- **Sclerotherapy** (injection therapy) uses sugar, salt or commercial sclerosing solutions to scar the veins, causing them to close off. You must be at least 12 weeks postpartum and not breastfeeding to have this treatment.
- **Surgical therapy** involves the tying off (ligation) of large veins to collapse the varicosed ones. Stripping is the removal of varicose veins by pulling them out of the legs.
- **Laser therapy** involves the use of a laser to cauterize (vaporize) varicose veins.

BREASTFEEDING
BREASTFEEDING BENEFITS

Mother

- Enhances maternal bonding.
- Provides a natural contraception (although not 100% effective).
- Speeds up the return to your pre-pregnancy weight (burns off an extra 500+ calories/day).
- Significant cost savings. Also saves time.
- Assists in the uterus returning to a normal size.
- Convenient, readily available and always the right temperature.
- Decreased risk of postpartum hemorrhage.
- Decreased risk of ovarian cancer.
- Decreased risk of premenopausal breast cancer.
- Decreased risk of osteoporosis.
- Causes a release of hormones that may assist in relaxation.
- Forces you to take regular breaks throughout the day.

Child

- Best-digested form of infant nutrition with the proper balance of nutrients, enzymes, antibodies and growth factors.
- Optimal nutritional delivery system.
- Breast milk changes to meet baby's maturing needs.
- Decreases the incidence of respiratory infections.
- Decreases the incidence of ear infections.
- Protects infant against allergic disorders and asthma.
- Reduces the chance of childhood obesity.
- May enhance intellectual and neurological development.
- Provides increased protection against diarrhea, colic, gas, spitting up and constipation.
- Enhances vaccine response.
- Decreases the incidence of SIDS (Sudden Infant Death Syndrome).
- Decreases the risk of type one (juvenile) diabetes.

Environmental/Health Concerns

- Reduces short-term and long-term healthcare costs.
- Environmentally friendly–less waste.
- Employer benefits–less sick time taken by parents.

BREASTFEEDING
10 SECRETS FOR SUCCESSFUL POSITIONING

NOTE: The "cross cradle" position will be highlighted as it is the easiest and allows for the most control with positioning.

1. Sit in a straight-backed, supportive chair. Use a footstool to elevate your feet. Sit in an upright position with relaxed shoulders. Do not lean forward into the baby.

2. Use a pillow that elevates the baby to the level of your breast and also support your arms.

3. Wear clothing that allows you easy access to the breasts. Have a drink and snack beside you while nursing.

4. Support your breast with a "C" or "U" hold by cupping your breast from underneath, with the thumb resting gently on the topside of the breast. Make sure all of your fingers are clear of the areola. (Photo A)

5. Position baby on a pillow so that their whole body is turned in to face your breast.

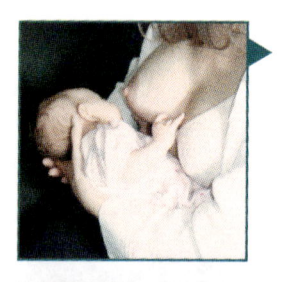

6. Support the baby's back with your forearm. With the palm of your hand supporting baby's neck and shoulders, grasp the baby's head (just behind or below the ears) on either side with your thumb and first or second finger.

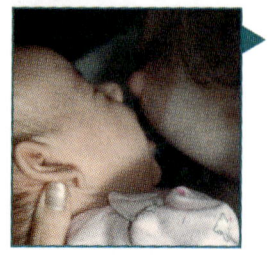

7. Align the baby so that the nipple is aimed between the nose and the upper lip. Do not use the mouth as a bull's-eye. The baby needs to "reach up" to the nipple.

Positioning and Latching Your Baby

130   YOUR HOME DOCTOR™ Mom

BREASTFEEDING
10 SECRETS FOR SUCCESSFUL POSITIONING

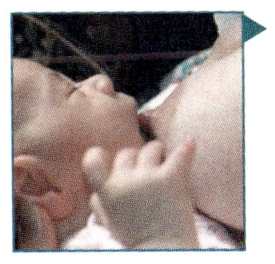

8. Stimulate the rooting reflex by rubbing the nipple on the baby's top lip and then move the baby away slightly. Wait until the baby opens mouth wide enough (like a yawn with the tongue down and out) before attempting to latch them. As you move the baby's head toward the breast, apply pressure with the palm of your hand (which is on the baby's shoulders/neck) so that the baby's head tilts slightly backwards. This will ensure that the chin and bottom lip will make first contact with the breast.

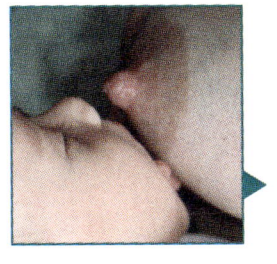

9. Catch the bottom lip about an inch away from the base of the nipple. By "catching" the bottom lip on the breast, the mouth is forced to open wider, allowing more breast to enter the baby's mouth. The top lip will land on the opposite side of the areola just above the nipple.

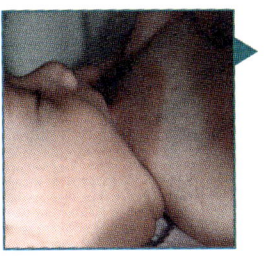

10. Keep the baby tucked in tightly to the breast to secure a wide-open latch. If you are worried about the baby's breathing, slide the baby's buttocks toward you with your elbow. This will bring baby's nose out and tuck the chin in even further.

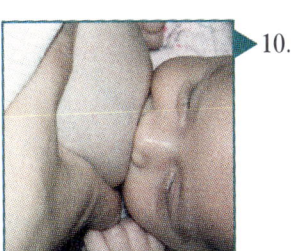

Positioning and Latching Your Baby

BREASTFEEDING
WHEN TO BREASTFEED (HUNGER CUES)

It is difficult to properly latch a screaming baby. The best time to latch is when they are showing early hunger cues. Get to know your baby's early hunger cues. Here are some common ones:

- Waking up, stirring and stretching.
- "Rooting" (turning head) toward breast with an open mouth.
- Licking their lips or sucking movements.
- Chewing on their fist or any nearby object.

Signs of a Good Latch

Babies who are "not getting enough milk" or who are jaundiced may not demonstrate these cues. See "Is Baby Getting Enough Milk?" and "Feeding the Sleepy Baby".

- Pain-free! A "fleeting tenderness" for a few seconds at the beginning of a feeding may be acceptable, but pain is your sign to unlatch your baby and try again.
- Baby will appear to have a "double chin." When their chin is pressed into the breast you will not see baby's lips.
- Baby's nose is resting on the breast, not "buried" in the breast.
- Baby's jaw movement with each suck moves their ears up and down.
- Gentle swallowing sounds are heard, progressing to gulping sounds as baby gets the "let down" of milk (gulping sounds may also be a quiet "eh" or "hee").
- You will see baby's Adam's apple or double chin move downward with each swallow. During let down, this should be at a 1:1 ratio of sucks to swallows. Mothers can have several let downs during a single feeding.

How to Unlatch a Baby

- A baby who has had a good feeding with plenty of good sucking and swallowing will come off by themselves at the end of the feed.
- To take the baby off the breast yourself (i.e., if you feel pain with latching), insert your forefinger or pinkie finger into the corner of the baby's mouth by sliding it alongside the breast far enough inside the mouth so that you hear a "popping" sound (the suction/vacuum seal is broken). Quickly slide the baby away from your nipple.

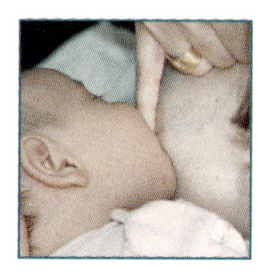

BREASTFEEDING
IS BABY GETTING ENOUGH MILK?

WARNING

**Take baby to your Doctor IMMEDIATELY
if baby is not demonstrating the following patterns:**

FEEDING

Day	1	2	3	4	5 and over
Number of Wet Diapers (voiding)	1	2	3	4	6 – 8
Number of Bowel Movements (stools)	1 (small)	2 (small)	3 (small)	4 (small)	1–2 large or 5 small
Bowel Movement (stool) Color	dark green or black and tarry (meconium)		transitional (changing from brown to yellow and seedy)		yellow and seedy

**Go to your Doctor IMMEDIATELY
if you have ANY of the following:**

- Baby feeds fewer than 8 to 12 times in a 24-hour period
- Baby is very sleepy. Baby may be either difficult to wake for feedings or fall asleep soon after being put to the breast.
- You are not hearing the baby swallowing. This sounds like an "eh" or "hee" during feedings.

SYMPTOMS

Infants will usually experience one or more of these signs
if not getting enough breastmilk during feedings:
- Appears hungry all the time (sucking on a fist or blanket)
- Appears irritable or cries soon after being taken off the breast
- Does not wake regularly for feedings. Babies, especially newborns, should wake at least every two to three hours.
- Falls asleep at breast early during a feed
- Does not demonstrate deep sucking and swallowing

GOALS

- To prevent baby losing more than 10% of birth weight during the first two weeks after delivery
- To return baby to birth weight by 2 to 3 weeks of age
- A weight gain in baby of approximately 1 oz. (28 grams) per day or 5 to 7 oz. (140 to 200 grams) per week up to 4 months of age and approximately 0.6 oz. (17 grams) per day after 4 months of age.

BREASTFEEDING
IS BABY GETTING ENOUGH MILK?

Trade Secrets

- Have baby weighed within the first two weeks after delivery.
- If concerned about how much your baby is getting, use the "Breastfeeding Record" on page 138 and compare to the chart under "Warnings" on the previous page.
- Watch for the signs of an improper latch: nipple soreness, cracking, blistering or bleeding, nipple compression (nipple looks flattened or compressed when it comes out of the baby's mouth) or whitening/blanching of the nipple tip. (See Latching Your Baby, page 130.)
- Babies who are feeding well and getting enough milk at breast will demonstrate the following feeding patterns:
    - After baby has latched on, a let down of milk occurs by baby suckling with very quick shallow sucks or a "quivering" movement
    - Once the milk lets down, baby's suck develops into a slow and steady deep suck (with jaw movement and ear "tugging" motion). There is a pause between baby's sucks, which is when the milk is being squirted into baby's mouth. The pause is followed by a swallow and a then a return to sucking.
    - During the feed there may be a number of "bursts" of deep sucking interspersed with a "nibbling" type of sucking.
    - Toward the end of the feed, there may be increasingly longer pauses between sucks, and the feed will end with the baby coming off the breast appearing satisfied.
    - It is important that a baby stays on the first breast as long as possible in order to ensure that baby is receiving the hindmilk before switching to the other breast.
- Jaundiced babies are at a higher risk for not getting enough because they are often more tired at the breast. Wake them every two to three hours to feed. They can have one long four to five hour sleep daily as long as they feed a minimum of 8 to 12 times per day.
- Babies often have growth spurts around 3 weeks, 6 weeks and 12 weeks. These usually last three to five days. Babies are often hungrier and fussy during these times. Feeding more often results in an increased milk production and a happier baby.
- When you feel supplementation is required, speak to your breastfeeding health professional. They can be invaluable in helping you with difficult feeding issues.

BREASTFEEDING
FEEDING THE SLEEPY BABY

WARNING
Go to your Doctor if you have ANY of the following:

- Doesn't seem to be getting enough milk • Is not stooling/urinating enough • Is not sucking/swallowing adequately • Is difficult to wake up for feeds • Is not feeding at least 8 to 12 times in a 24-hour period • Develops a fever • Develops signs of jaundice (skin and/or whites of the eyes turn yellow) • Looks or acts sick

SYMPTOMS
- Baby falls asleep soon after going to breast
- Baby is difficult to wake or sleeps long periods throughout the day without waking for feeds • Baby feeds less than 8 to 12 times in a 24-hour period.

GOALS
To learn how to stimulate a sleepy baby and to monitor and ensure an adequate intake of milk. This section generally refers to babies less than four months old.

TIPS
- Many medications, including herbal, have sedating effects on babies. Beware of all medication taken by you or given to baby.
- In hospital, room in with your new baby so feedings can be frequent and you can learn how to recognize your infant's early feeding cues.
- Early feeding cues normally include: stirring and stretching, "rooting" (turning their head toward the breast with an open mouth), licking their lips or sucking movements, chewing on their fist or any nearby objects.
- Beware of pacifiers, which may tire your baby out for breastfeeding. They may also mask the true signs of hunger.
- If supplements are medically necessary, try cup feeding, finger feeding or lactation aids at breast if you are concerned about maintaining breastfeeding. Speak to your breastfeeding health professional for help with these methods.
- Waking baby every two to three hours may be necessary early on to ensure adequate feeds. Allow baby one to two long naps a day to satisfy their deep sleep needs.
- 8 to 12 feeds are necessary in a 24-hour period.
- Read "Is Baby Getting Enough Milk?" (pg. 133).

YOUR HOME DOCTOR™ Mom

BREASTFEEDING
FEEDING THE SLEEPY BABY

Use the following tips to wake baby up or to keep baby awake during feeds.

- Undress baby to diaper and feed "skin to skin."
- Change the diaper before switching to the second side.
- Talk to your baby throughout the feeding.
- Stroke the spine, hands, soles of baby's feet or under the chin.
- Express some breastmilk onto the baby's lips.
- Wipe the baby's face with a cool damp cloth.
- Encourage continued feeding with breast compression.

Breast Compression (Massage)

Breast compression is used to:
- Stimulate mother's milk let down
- Increase mother's milk flow
- Encourage baby's continued sucking and swallowing
- Check for and break-up plugged milk ducts

Breast compression is performed as follows:

1) Free one of your arms while breastfeeding. Support baby's head with one hand.
2) Cup the feeding breast with your other hand, thumb on one side, fingers on the other side, but keep your fingers clear of the areola.
3) When baby's sucking slows or when baby begins to fall asleep at breast, compress (squeeze) the breast. It should not hurt when you compress, and the shape of the areola should not change.
4) Hold this squeezing action until the baby stops sucking and swallowing, then release the breast.
5) If baby continues to suck and swallow after the breast is released, do not compress again. If baby's sucking and swallowing decrease again, try compressing again.
6) Continue this process until baby fails to suck and swallow even when the compression action is applied.

BREASTFEEDING
BREASTFEEDING RECORD

Introduction

The Breastfeeding Record can be used by parents to monitor how their baby is feeding and whether their baby is getting enough milk. It is also helpful to have this record available when consulting a breastfeeding health professional, so that accurate feeding, urine and stooling information can be shared.

Using the Breastfeeding Record

Date

Time

Length of time "deep sucking" and swallowing
(Left / Right Breast)
When a baby first goes to the breast they begin to suck and a let down is initiated. Baby then begins a slow and steady "deep" suck (you will see jaw movement or ear tugging). With this type of suck, there is a definite pause between the baby's sucks (or compression of the breast) that results in the milk being squirted into baby's mouth. The pause is immediately followed by a swallow. Mothers will sometimes hear their babies swallow by making a little "hee" sound. This column records how long the baby actually "deep" sucks and swallows.

Total Time at Breast
(Left / Right Breast)
This column records the total time (in minutes) that baby is spending on each breast from the beginning to the end of a feeding.

Disposition After Feeding
This records how baby appears when finished the feed (e.g., fell asleep at breast, fell off breast, came off crying, alert, etc.) and how baby acted a short while after the feed (e.g., napped for 20 minutes, was fussy 15 minutes after the feed, gassy, etc.).

Urine
This column records the number of wet diapers and the amount the diaper was wet: 1. (small), 2. (medium) or 3. (large).

Stool
This column records the number of bowel movements and whether amounts were: 1. (small), 2. (medium) or 3. (large). Color (black and tarry, brown or yellow) and consistency (watery, soft, pasty or hard) are also recorded here.

BREASTFEEDING
BREASTFEEDING RECORD

Date	Time	Length of Time Deep swallow Left | Right	Total Time at Breast Left | Right	Disposition After Feeding	Urine	Stools

The Breastfeeding Record

BREASTFEEDING
PUMPING BREASTMILK

Why Pump?

- To increase mother's milk supply.
- If a baby is unable to latch and feed at breast.
- When mother is unable to be with baby (such as when infant hospitalized for prematurity).
- To relieve engorgement or to soften breast enough for the baby to latch well.
- To store breastmilk (especially for a mother who is going out or returning to work or school).

When Would you Pump?

- The best time of day to pump is in the morning, when milk production is highest. The worst time to pump is in the evening, when production is lowest.
- Remember, the amount obtained by pumping IS NOT indicative of how much the baby is getting.
- The best time to pump is when the baby is feeding on the other side and the let down has started.

Stimulating Your Let Down Before Pumping

- Release of the hormone oxytocin, which controls milk let down, is influenced by physical and psychological triggers such as specific sounds, smells and touches.
- Some mothers' oxytocin release, and therefore milk let down, cannot be stimulated by using mechanical devices such as breast pumps.

Tips to Help with Let Down

- Express your milk in a relaxed place without distractions.
- Express at approximately the same time every day.
- Follow this pre-pumping routine:
  a) Wash your hands.
  b) Apply low heat to breasts 15 minutes before pumping. Use warm compress, a hot water bottle or a heating pad.
  c) Gently massage your breasts.
  d) Stimulate your nipples by rolling them between the thumb and forefinger.
  e) Relax for 5 minutes (take a few deep breaths and think about a calming scene before focusing on the pleasant image of your baby).

BREASTFEEDING
PUMPING BREASTMILK

Methods of Pumping

There are two ways that a mother can pump her breasts:

- Hand expression
- With a breast pump

HAND EXPRESSION

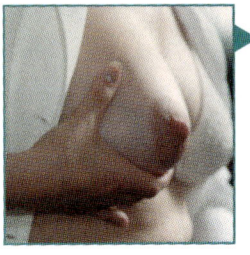

STEP #1
- Cup the breast in a C–hold.

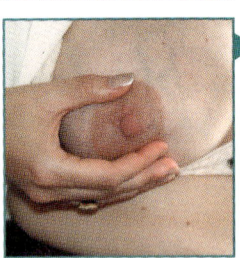

STEP #2
- Feel for your milk ducts (they will feel like little grape clusters under the skin, usually at the outer edge of the areola).
- Place your thumb and forefinger over the top of your ducts.

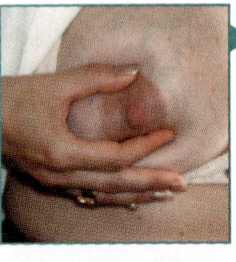

STEP #3
- Press straight back toward your chest.

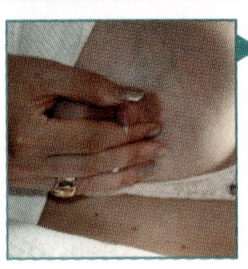

STEP #4
- Keeping your fingers still, compress your thumb and forefinger together while you roll fingers over the ducts.

STEP #5
- Return to step 3. As you rotate around your breast (imagine your breast is like a clock), express the hours of the clock.

BREASTFEEDING
PUMPING BREASTMILK

BREAST PUMPS

Manual Pumps (Egnell Ameda or Medela)

- Easy to use, portable, small, easy to clean, inexpensive.
- Are appropriate for occasional outings or pumpings.
- Are cylinder pumps that require two hands to operate.
- The Egnell Ameda one-hand pump requires one hand to operate and can be used to pump while the baby is feeding on the other side.

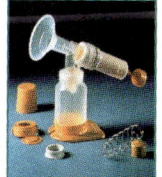

Spring Express™ Manual Pump

Mini Electric Pumps

- Allows mother to control the suction and rhythm of pumping.
- Convenient (faster and easier to carry).
- Only takes one hand to operate the pump. Allows you to pump on one side while the baby feeds on the other.
- Appropriate for more regular pumping or when returning to work while trying to maintain your milk supply.

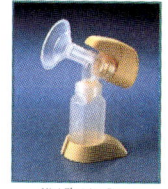

Mini-Electric™ Pump

Electric Rental Pumps

- Recommended for special circumstances requiring early or frequent pumping (e.g., a premature infant).
- Allows for double pumping, which increases milk supply and cuts down on pumping time.
- Daily rental fee and fee for the pumping kit.
- The pumping kit can be converted into a manual pump by purchasing the handle attachment.

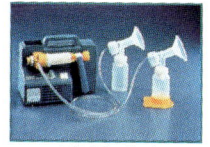

Lactina™ BreastPump

Breast pump photos courtesy of Medela® Canada Inc.

Pumping Times

- Double Pumping–10 minutes total.
- Single Pumping–5 minutes per side and repeat (20 minutes total).

Note: Stop pumping when the milk is no longer flowing (which may be earlier than the prescribed time).

Pumping Tips

- Read the instructions for use and cleaning.
- Always wash your hands before pumping.
- Use the flange/cup insert that best fits your breast. A good pump will accommodate breast size differences by including a flange.
- Always begin pumping on a low setting. Gradually increase the pressure of the pump depending upon your comfort level.
- Pain indicates the need to change to the other breast or to adjust the pump pressure.

YOUR HOME DOCTOR™ Mom

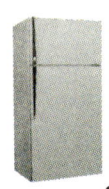

BREASTFEEDING
STORING BREASTMILK

What Do I Store the Milk In?

- Glass is the best type of container to store breastmilk in. It is the least likely to affect the properties of breastmilk (try glass baby bottles or a small jam/mason jar).
- Hard plastic containers should be your second choice. Ensure the container is new or cleaned well and without scratches.
- Soft plastic bags are not recommended as they are fragile, easily punctured and difficult to create an airtight seal in. An airtight seal is essential when storing milk.
- Write the date and time of milk collection on the container.

Tips for Storing Milk

	Room Temp.	Refrigerator	Fridge/Freezer	Deep Freezer (−19°C)
Freshly Pumped Breastmilk	4–8 hours	5–8 days	2 weeks (freezer inside fridge) 3–4 months (freezer with separate door)	6 months
Thawed Breastmilk (from freezer)	Do not store at this temperature	24 hours (It is better to serve thawed breastmilk immediately)	Do not refreeze breastmilk	Do not refreeze breastmilk

- Don't refrigerate expressed breastmilk if it is to be used within eight hours.
- Chill expressed breastmilk in the refrigerator before freezing.
- You can add two fresh or refrigerated pumpings together if they are to be served right away.
- Thaw frozen or refrigerated milk by placing the container under cool running water and then gradually increasing the temperature of the water until it reaches body temperature (37°C or 98.5°F). Heating above 60°C (140°F) may destroy some of the properties of breastmilk.
- Never microwave breastmilk. It destroys breastmilk properties.
- Store expressed breastmilk in different amounts (2, 4, 6 oz.) depending on the amount the baby is consuming. In this way, if baby is still hungry after a feeding, another 2 or 4 oz. may be offered without wasting your breastmilk supplies.
- Discard any unused milk after feeding baby.
- Thawed breastmilk can be refrigerated for up to 24 hours (but do not refreeze).

BREASTFEEDING
FEEDING YOUR BABY WHEN YOU ARE AWAY

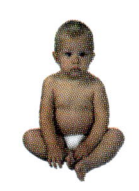

There are many feeding options for mothers to consider when they have to be away from their baby. Breastfeeding, supplementing, cup feeding, formula feeding, and introduction of solids and juices all need to be thought over. Consider some of these important issues:

Baby Concerns

- It is not advisable to introduce a bottle before the baby's latch at breast is well established (at least four weeks of age). This is to lessen the chance of "nipple confusion."
- An older baby (six weeks or older) can be introduced to a bottle or cup for use during a mother's absence.
- The easiest way to supplement or feed a baby without introducing a bottle is using cup feeding. Speak to your breastfeeding health professional for advice regarding this.
- Always feed baby early when they first exhibit "hunger cues."
(See When to breastfeed page 132). It is always easier to feed a baby if they are not fussing or screaming with hunger.
- When using alternative forms of feeding it is helpful to place baby in a feeding position different from the breastfeeding position.

Separation Concerns

- Mothers who return to work or school may be able to continue breastfeeding, with the baby taking solids, juices and water while the mother is away, and still feeding three to four times when mother returns home.
- Mothers returning to work or school may find their babies do not want formula but would rather "catch up" on breastfeeding upon mother's return (depending on the length of mother's absence and the age of the child).
- Mothers having long absences from their baby may consider pumping and storing breastmilk for their baby. (See Pumping Breastmilk, page 140, and Storing Breastmilk, page 142.)
- During long absences from their babies, mothers may choose to supplement their baby with expressed breastmilk or formula.
- Whatever method of feeding you choose, have someone else introduce it first. You will also likely need to leave the room in order for baby to feed cooperatively.
- When introducing a bottle to a breastfed baby, use an oversized orthodontic nipple (not the newborn size). Slightly warm the nipple before use.

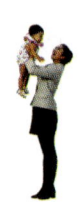

BREASTFEEDING
FEEDING YOUR BABY WHEN YOU ARE AWAY

Childcare Concerns

- How a mother feeds her baby while separated from her infant is often dependent on the childcare arrangements.
- Introduce your baby to the childcare provider several times before returning to work or school to help in the transition.
- If choosing cup feeding, make sure your caregiver is taught how ahead of time and is thoroughly comfortable with it.
- Share helpful hints and techniques in feeding your baby with your childcare provider. This helps to make the transition in feeding a smooth one and easier for baby.

Milk Supply Concerns

- Concerns about milk supply often depend upon the length of time away and how supportive the workplace and employer are to breastfeeding and/or pumping on work breaks and during lunch.
- Mother may need to supplement baby with an additional feeding of solids and/or formula when her milk supply starts to decline.
(See Weaning Your Baby, page 145.)

Return to Work/School Concerns

- Get baby used to the childcare provider before returning to work or school. Make sure your childcare provider is comfortable with your chosen method of feeding your baby.
- Get baby used to a bottle or cup before your first absence.
- If breastfeeding try to maintain six to eight weeks of uninterrupted breastfeeding before returning to work or school.
- If supplementing with breastmilk is planned, start to accumulate a supply of frozen breastmilk at least two weeks before returning to work or school.
- Try to return to work or school on a Thursday or Friday to give you a short week and thereby help to maintain your strength and energy. This will also allow you time to solve problems over the weekend.
- Wear clothing that are easy to breastfeed in. These may include printed blouses, jackets and sweaters to conceal leaking. To stop leaking, apply firm pressure to your breast by pressing the nipple back into the breast. Use washable cotton breast pads to protect your clothing.

BREASTFEEDING
WEANING YOUR BABY

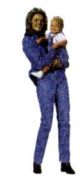

General Tips On Weaning

- Weaning is a process of reducing or discontinuing breastfeeding.
- Weaning is most effective when it is a gradual process.
- Gradual weaning minimizes breast problems and provides an easier adjustment for baby and mom.
- Breastfeeding challenges often lead to early weaning. These problems can often be resolved and breastfeeding continued (if so desired) by consulting a breastfeeding health professional. Problems might include:
  – Maternal illness including mastitis
  – Mother taking medication or requiring diagnostic tests
  – New pregnancy
  – Teething baby
  – Extremely painful nipples
  – Return to work or school
  – Concern that baby is not getting enough milk

Since weaning can be an emotional process, support is essential. If a mother is concerned about the weaning process, she should talk to a breastfeeding health professional. The La Leche League is also an excellent resource on breastfeeding and weaning.

HOW TO WEAN
Gradual Weaning
(Slowing Down to a Stop)

- This method is used to stop breastfeeding completely.
- Eliminate one breastfeeding (usually the same feeding) per day every three to five days. If going back to work, plan ahead and begin weaning two to three weeks before your work start date.
- Feeds can be replaced with cup feeding or bottle feeding and/or solids, depending on the baby's age.
- Sometimes babies or toddlers will "naturally" and gradually wean themselves from the breast.
- Certain behaviors may indicate that weaning is progressing too fast: night-waking, biting, negative behaviors, separation anxiety, clinging to mother or attachment to an object (some children turn to an alternative sucking such as thumb sucking, bottle or pacifiers).

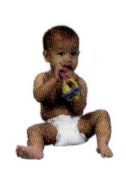

BREASTFEEDING
WEANING YOUR BABY

Partial Weaning
(Slowing Down with No Stop)

- Great for returning to work and wanting to breastfeed only for one nighttime feed.
- Like gradual weaning this method needs to be done slowly, so that milk supply does not drop too suddenly.
- Involves consistently dropping one nursing (e.g., afternoon nursing) or nursings (as though the baby were beginning to wean) while continuing to breastfeed the rest of the feeds.
- Partial weaning may be performed over a short or long term.
- You may return to full nursing at your discretion.
- Certain behaviors may indicate that weaning is progressing too fast. (See Gradual Weaning).

Abrupt Weaning
(Sudden Stop)

- The most difficult method for mother and baby.
- Usually performed because of a sudden problem.
- Mother and baby may experience emotional strain.
- Mother may experience severe engorgement and mastitis.
- Follow the treatment for engorgement (see Breast Engorgement, pg. 33). Reduce the pumping frequency. If the baby had been feeding every two to three hours, pump every three to four hours and slowly increase to longer periods between pumpings.

Baby-Led Weaning
(Natural Stop)

- This method allows the child to develop and achieve independence from breastfeeding at their own pace.
- Extends the health benefits of breastfeeding for the child and mother.
- Mother may need to consider ways to avoid the social stigma of breastfeeding an older child in public. You may want to use a code word for breastfeeding that others will not recognize. In this way you can communicate effectively with your child when they are asking to breastfeed in public.

BOTTLE FEEDING
BOTTLE FEEDING BENEFITS

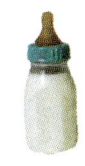

Mother

- No vaginal dryness or loss of libido.
- No engorged or leaking breasts.
- No sore, cracked nipples, breast or nipple pain.
- Reduced incidence of mastitis.
- No problems with latching, pain or "nipple confusion."
- No difficulty with insufficient milk production.
- More choices for birth control.
- Easier to keep track of baby's milk intake.
- More feeding help possible by others (partner, grandparents, etc). This is especially important when mom is exhausted, sick, or is not the primary caregiver.
- Easier to return to work outside the home. Increased freedom is possible. This may be especially important to professional women or those who need to travel a lot.
- Fewer nutritional demands on the body.
- No need to pump or express milk.
- No restrictions on diet, medications or vitamin therapies.
- Fewer public or workplace feeding problems.
- Helpful for those with fertility concerns, those who are trying to conceive, or those on fertility agents.
- Helpful for those who have had previous breast surgery, radiation treatment or physical handicaps.
- Sometimes helpful in severe cases of postpartum depression or in cases of postpartum psychosis.
- A useful choice for mothers with various medical, psychiatric or emotional concerns.

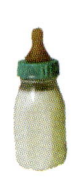

BOTTLE FEEDING
BOTTLE FEEDING BENEFITS

Child

- May feel full for longer periods of time. This may result in longer periods between feedings.
- Safety from medicines, viruses, toxins or other chemicals passed from mother. This is most important with mothers addicted to drugs or alcohol. This is also important with mothers who must take medications.
- Supplementation often necessary for low–birthweight babies.
- Helpful in babies with failure to thrive.
- May be necessary for babies with latch or suck difficulties or mouth or tongue problems, including a cleft lip or palate.
- Often necessary for children of multiple births.
- May be necessary in cases of severe infant jaundice.
- No sensitivities resulting from mother's diet.
- Useful when baby has severe allergies to milk sugar or milk protein.

BOTTLE FEEDING

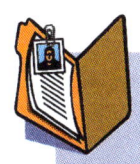

CASE STUDY

Mary Ann came to the office two weeks postpartum. I asked how her breastfeeding was going.

"Well, I tried the breastfeeding but I just didn't like it," she said. "Since then I've put Samantha on formula and both of us are much happier. Even my husband is happier. He's thrilled that he can now give her a bottle as well. I know I will take some flak from my friends for not breastfeeding, but I really am happier. Is there anything I need to know about the types of formula, bottles or anything else that would help me with my decision? Are there any dangers involved with bottle feeding?"

Mary Ann and I spent the next 15 minutes discussing the ins and outs of bottle feeding formula.

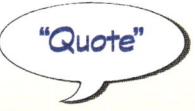

"Quote"

Freedom of choice means never having to say you are sorry for not breastfeeding.

Guilt does nothing to satisfy your baby's hunger.

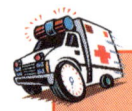

BOTTLE FEEDING

WARNING
Go to your Doctor IMMEDIATELY if your baby has ANY of the following:
- Seems constantly unhappy or hungry • Not taking formula
- Does not seem to be gaining weight
- Not having one bowel movement and six wet diapers per day
- Passing hard dry stool • Passing black stools
- Mucus or blood in the stool • Inactive and lethargic

DEFINITION
Bottle feeding can be of two types, with or without associated breastfeeding. Bottled formula can be used as the main source of nutrition or used to supplement breastfed infants.

GOALS
To provide appropriate nutrition and promote normal growth and development.

TIPS
- Ask your doctor to recommend a formula or to assist you in changing a formula because of an intolerance by baby.
- Make bottle feeding, like breastfeeding, a special time. Take your time, talk and touch your baby as you feed.
- It is never recommended to heat milk in a microwave. Heat in warm water and shake well before giving the bottle to a baby.
- Specialty formulas are used for specific infant nutrition needs. Speak to your doctor before starting one.
- Ignore the negative comments you encounter. Guilt has no nutritional value in the feeding of your child. A happy, healthy baby and mother is the only goal of importance.
- Milk and soy-based formulas are the main formula choices.
- Milk-based formulas are used for the majority of infants.
- Soy-based formulas or milk-based but lactose-free formulas are used for infants with milk intolerance or allergies and when treating babies with diarrhea/vomiting (gastroenteritis).
- A switch to another formula may help infants with excessive gas, vomiting, abdominal cramps, diarrhea or skin rashes.
- Sterilize bottles and nipples daily until baby is four months old.
- When supplementing with formula, always breastfeed first. When you feel baby has received all they can at breast, then give them the bottle. Keep track of how much formula they take.
- Burp between breast and bottle or halfway through the bottle. Newborns need to be burped every 1 to 1 1/2 oz.
- Newborn babies often need to be fed small amounts frequently.
- Never force baby to feed or to finish a bottle.

BOTTLE FEEDING

READ WARNING

Are you supplementing breastfeeding?

Yes:
- Breastfeed first from both breasts.
- Supplement with 2 to 4 oz. of formula.
- Record the amount taken at each feeding.
- See your doctor regularly to evaluate baby's weight gain and development.
- Sterilize nipples and bottles for the first four months.

No:
- Newborn babies usually take 2 to 4 oz. every 2 to 4 hours.
- Older babies will take more milk and last longer between feedings.
- Learn to watch for signs of baby getting full (turns head away, loses interest, stops sucking).
- Burp baby halfway through a feeding.
- Try different nipples and bottles to find which one baby prefers.
- Place baby in a reclining or sitting position, not lying down.
- Try different formulas to determine baby's preference.
- Speak to your doctor before you add solid foods.
- Do not bottle feed in cribs.
- Sterilize nipples and bottles for the first four months.

Is your baby active, alert, and content?

- **Yes:** Continue with present feeding plan.
- **No:** Go to Doctor.

BOTTLE FEEDING

Trade Secrets

- Bottle feeding mothers are often looked down upon as second-class parents. The guilt and influence that this can place on a new mother is enormous. However, for some women breastfeeding is not a reasonable option. If you choose not to breastfeed, hold your head up high, choose a good formula and know that your child will still turn out just fine.
- Most commercial formulas in North America are nutritionally similar, as they all must conform to a stringent set of national nutritional and component guidelines.
- Soy-based formulas (made from soya beans) often give babies bad breath and foul-smelling stools.
- Cow's milk is great for calves but is not ideal for human babies.
- Infants can be safely switched from milk-based formulas to cow's milk around 12 to 14 months of age.
- Formula-fed infants need 2 to 2.5 oz. (55 to 70 ml.) per pound of body weight per day. Therefore, a 10 lb. child will need 20 to 25 oz. (550 to 700 ml.) of formula per day. Babies under four months of age normally gain about 5 to 7 oz./week (or 140 to 200 grams/week).
- Powdered formula is usually the most economical way to purchase formula. Concentrates and ready-to-use formulas are easier to make but more expensive to buy.
- Mix powdered formula carefully to keep the strength consistent.
- Never allow baby to fall asleep with a bottle propped in their mouth.
- Feed baby in a reclining position, not when lying flat.

Definitions

- **Bottle feeding** is synonymous with formula feeding. However, it can be supplemental bottle feeding to a breastfed infant.
- **Hypoallergenic formulas** (Nutramigen, Alimentum, Soyalac).
- **Lactose-free formulas** (Enfalac lactose free, Similac LF).
- **Milk-based formulas** (Enfalac, Similac, Unilac, Good Start, SMA).
- **Soy-based formulas** (ProSobee, Isomil).
- **Specialty formulas** include those for infants with impaired digestion or absorption as well as thickened or next-step formulas.
- **Gastroenteritis** is a bowel infection that causes vomiting and/or diarrhea

Synonyms

- Formula feeding • Supplemental feeding.

Medications/Treatments

- **Types of formula** include ready-to-use, concentrate and powder. They are a balance between convenience and cost.

POSTPARTUM CHECKUP

This is normally performed at around six weeks after delivery. Traumatic or cesarean section births are usually seen sooner.

What to Expect

The Physical Exam

- Height, weight and blood pressure check.
- An examination of the size and shape of your uterus. This is to make sure it is returning to a pre-pregnancy size.
- Assessment of healing in the vagina including checking tears and episiotomy sites as well as the pelvic floor muscles.
- A check of the cervix, including a Pap smear.
- Evaluation of your bladder function. This includes a urine dip test to check for infection.
- Evaluation of your bowel function including checking your hemorrhoids, if you have them.
- A breast examination.
- An assessment for swelling in the legs and varicose veins.
- Checkup of any muscle pain or joint instability. This includes any back difficulties.
- Remember to ask your doctor to check for diastasis recti (separation of the stomach muscles) before starting back to exercising. If present you will need special stomach exercises to bring them together again.

The Psychological Exam

A discussion about:
- Postpartum blues or depression symptoms. This may also include taking a postpartum depression questionnaire.
- Support at home and in the community.
- Coping strategies.
- The delivery and motherhood. Do you have any dissappointments? or do you have any regrets?
- Any relationship difficulties (partner, other children, etc.).
- Current sleep and feeding schedules.
- A return-to-work plan.
- Breastfeeding progress and future plans.

Birth control should be discussed at this visit.

Bring a list of all your health questions to the checkup.

COPING

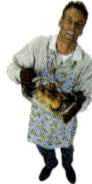

YOUR FIRST DAYS AT HOME

After the build-up of your pregnancy, the physical demands of the delivery and the elation of seeing your new baby, you may suddenly begin to feel the magnitude of your new responsibility once it's time to take the baby home. After all, you are sent home from hospital with this new, fragile, little person who looks to you for the satisfaction of all their worldly needs. Feel overwhelmed? You don't need to be if you have a plan. Here are tips to help you organize your life and better prepare you for the roller-coaster ride of your upcoming first year.

Things to do

- PRIORITIZE but don't put yourself last!
- Focus on one day at a time and one task at a time. Keep daily goals attainable and expect plenty of interruptions.
- If you don't have help, get some. When people offer to help, accept and put them to work on things that would most benefit you. This usually means laundry, housecleaning, cooking, grocery shopping, errands or other chores. Consider hiring a housecleaning service to help you out.
- Use the frozen dinners you received from friends, family or purchased at the grocery store.
- Rest when your baby does. Ignore your guilt and just do it.
- Use the answering machine to screen calls. Leave a message on the machine that you are busy with your new baby and will call back as soon as you are able.
- Get help from a certified lactation consultant or the La Leche League if you are having any trouble breastfeeding.
- Learn to develop and rely on your parents' intuition.
- Get showered and dressed before your partner leaves for work. Your partner can watch the baby while you get prepared.
- Wear comfortable, washable clothing. Breastmilk and baby stains do not dry clean well.
- Stockpile supplies: buy double diaper packs, wipes, formula, laundry soap.
- Read Baby Blues. It's a great comic strip for new parents. Always remember to keep your sense of humor!

Things not to do

- Anything that does not revolve around you or the baby. This includes dinner parties for twelve, yard work or anything vaguely resembling exercise. There will be plenty of time for these things later.

154   YOUR HOME DOCTOR™ Mom

COPING

YOUR FIRST WEEKS AT HOME

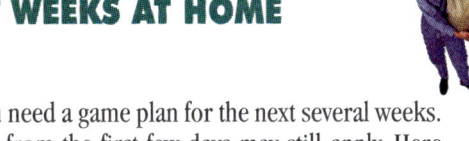

Once things start to settle down, you need a game plan for the next several weeks. Some of the same do's and don'ts from the first few days may still apply. Here are some other things to consider.

Things to do

- PRIORITIZE but don't put yourself last!
- Focus on one day and one task at a time. Keep your expectations reasonable and expect more interruptions.
- Continue to rest when your baby rests.
- Eat small, healthy snacks frequently. Drink water and juices.
- Limit the number of visitors during the first month.
- Don't expect any routine until at least six weeks postpartum.
- Expect the unexpected. Allow time for spit-ups, diaper changes, accidents and days of chaos.
- Use lists to assist you with postpartum forgetfulness.
- Allow your partner to learn how to parent too. Increase their time alone with baby, allow them to share nighttime duties and general care duties. Overlook their small mistakes.
- Learn together and have fun. Parenting is a team sport.
- Save time shopping–buy in bulk (large supplies).
- Consider using mail-order catalogues for purchases.
- Fill out your baby book while awaiting doctor's appointments.
- Get out of the house at least 30 minutes each day.
- Do a load of wash every morning and/or evening.
- Stay flexible and reconsider your expectations (e.g. what is a clean house?). You and your baby should remain the first priority.
- Prepare diaper bag, formula and clothes for next day in the evening when baby goes to sleep. Twenty minutes of efficiency today will save you an hour of chaos tomorrow.
- Remember, new babies are often unsettled for two to four hours per day and approximately one day per week. This is NORMAL.
- Start exercising even if it's just a daily walk with baby.
- Find routines and a division of labor that work for all the members of your growing family. All families are unique.
- Remember to spend time with your partner.
- Keep your sense of humor!
- When returning to work, ease in slowly, trying half days or returning midweek. This will allow both baby and you some time to adjust to your additional work demands.

"We are what we repeatedly do." – Aristotle

BIRTH CONTROL

Method	How It Works	Strengths
Barrier Methods		
Condom	Prevents entry of sperm into the cervix	Reversible, non-invasive, HIV and STD prevention
Spermicide	Kills sperm in the vagina	Reversible
Sponge	Same as condom and spermicide	Safe to use when breastfeeding, reversible
Diaphragm	Same as condom	Non-invasive, reversible, safe to use when breastfeeding
The Pill		
Progesterone–only Pill	Prevents ovulation, makes uterus unfavorable for pregnancy, decreases sperm migration	Effective, reversible, safe when breastfeeding, less menstrual flow and cramping, less pelvic inflammatory disease, fewer ovarian cysts
Combination Pill	Same as above	Same as above except not advised in breastfeeding (may decrease milk supply)
Injections		
Progesterone	Prevents ovulation	Easier to remember–only need injection every 3 months

BIRTH CONTROL

Weaknesses	Contraindications	Effectiveness
Barrier Methods		
Latex allergies, breakage	Allergies (latex)	88–98%
Reliability varies, less spontaneity, manual application is unappealing to some	Allergies	79–97%
Same as above, Toxic Shock risk	Allergies	72–94%
May dislodge, less spontaneity, manual application unappealing to some, diaphragm needs resizing when weight changes ≥ 15 lb.	Allergies	82–94%
The Pill		
Breakthrough bleeding, nausea, breast tenderness, clotting risks, appetite changes, can affect the liver, can interact with other medications	Smoker older than 35, hypertension, clotting risk, breast cancer, liver disease, migraine headaches	97–99.5%
Same as above	Same as above	97–99.9%
Injections		
Nausea, headaches, irregular periods, mood changes, weight gain, breast tenderness, delay in return to fertility, decrease in bone density	Liver disease, clotting risks, breast cancer, depression	99.7%

BIRTH CONTROL

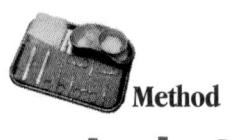

Method	How It Works	Strengths
Implants		
Norplant	Prevents ovulation	Good for 5 year (cannot forget to take or use), safety during breastfeeding not proven
IUD		
	Makes uterus unfavorable to sperm, may prevent implantation of fertilized egg	Effective for 3 years, inexpensive, convenient, safe with breastfeeding
Surgery		
Vasectomy	Blocks sperm	Local anesthetic, simple office procedure, less invasive than tubal ligation, one-time procedure, effective, permanent
Tubal Ligation	Blocks egg access to the uterus	One-time procedure, effective, permanent
Others		
Abstinence	Prevention	Non-invasive
Rhythm	Identifying and avoiding sex during high-risk (fertile) times in the cycle	Non-invasive, reversible, no pills, needles or devices required

BIRTH CONTROL

Weaknesses	Contraindications	Effectiveness

Implants

Infection and itching, removal difficulty, irregular periods, increase in ovarian cysts frequency, initial cost, headache, hair loss, abdominal discomfort.	Liver disease, clotting risks, breast cancer, depression	99.7%

IUD

Pregnancy at risk if conceived with IUD in, heavier periods usually with increased cramping, risk of infection or perforation, unnoticed IUD expulsion (rare)	Copper allergy, fibroids, vaginal infection	97–99%

Surgery

Reluctance of partner, local tenderness, poor reversibility if more than after surgery, infection and bleeding risk, invasive, expense of reversing, risk of failure (rare)	Bleeding risk, uncertainty about wanting the procedure done	99.8%
Invasive, general anesthetic risk, infection and bleeding risk, may increase menstrual cramps, expense of reversing, risk of failure (rare)	Bleeding or anesthetic risk, uncertainty about wanting the procedure done	99.6%

Others

Needs high motivation	None	100%
Confusion if menstrual cycles irregular or unpredictable, poor reliability, time consuming procedures increase accuracy, needs high motivation	None	80–91%

NUTRITION AND VITAMINS
Daily Food Pyramid

General Nutrition Guidelines
- Eat a variety of foods.
- Maintain a healthy weight.
- Choose a diet low in fat, especially saturated fats and cholesterol.
- Eat many vegetables, fruits, and grain products.
- Use sugar and salt (sodium) in moderation.
- Eat foods as close to their natural state as possible.

Fats, Oils, Sweets
Use sparingly

Milk, Yogurt, Cheese
2–3 Servings

Meat, Poultry, Fish, Eggs, Nuts
2–3 Servings

Vegetables
3–5 Servings

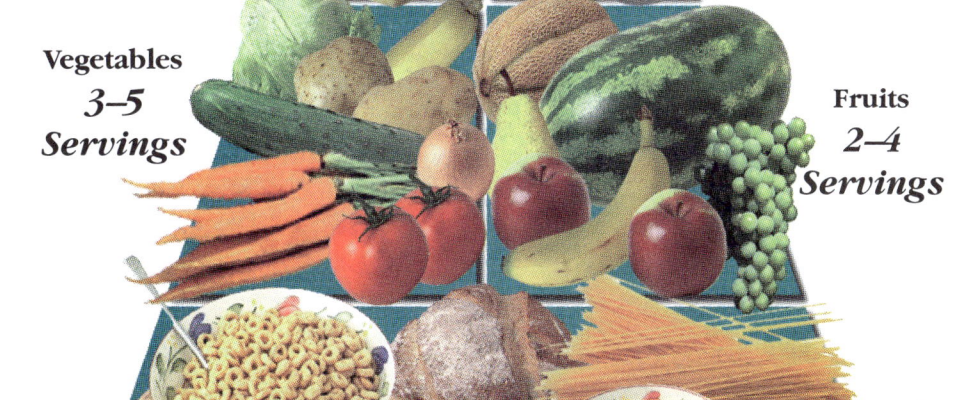

Fruits
2–4 Servings

Bread, Cereal, Rice, Pasta
6–11 Servings

Daily Food Pyramid

YOUR HOME DOCTOR™ Mom

IMPORTANT NUTRIENTS

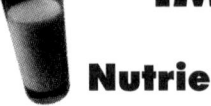

Nutrient	Food Source	What It Does
Carbohydrates	Bread, cereal, fruit, pasta, potatoes, rice, sugar	Provide energy
Fats and oils	Butter, cheese, margarine, meats, nuts, oils, salad dressing	Provide energy and help absorb fat soluble vitamins
Milk products	Butter, cheese, milk, yogurt	Build and maintain bones and teeth
Protein	Cheese, eggs, fish, nuts, tofu, legume's, meat, milk	Builds and repairs body tissues

MINERALS

Nutrient	Food Source	What It Does
Calcium	Milk and milk products, salmon, sardines, oysters, nuts, tofu	Builds and maintains bones and teeth, also important for muscle and nerve function
Iodine	Salt and seafoods (crab, lobster, shrimp)	Important for thyroid gland function
Iron	Iron-enriched breads and cereals, organ and red meats, dried fruits	Important component of oxygen-carrying red blood cells
Magnesium	Beef, liver, nuts, grains, shellfish	Builds and maintains bones and teeth and needed for tissue production
Phosphorus	Milk and milk products, breads, meat, nuts	Builds and maintains bones and teeth
Zinc	Eggs, meat, nuts, shellfish, fish, whole grains and seeds	Tissue production, healing and energy breakdown

IMPORTANT NUTRIENTS

Nutrient   Food Source   What It Does

VITAMINS

Nutrient	Food Source	What It Does
Vitamin A	Liver, apricots, carrots, peppers, sweet potatoes, spinach, squash	Maintains healthy skin, bones and teeth, aids in night vision
Vitamin B1 (Thiamine)	Brewer's yeast, wheat germ, beans, nuts, peas	Helps metabolize carbohydrates needed for growth
Vitamin B2 (Riboflavin)	Brewer's yeast, organ meats, wheat germ, wild rice, egg yolks, mushrooms	For healthy skin, eyes, nervous system
Vitamin B3 (Niacin)	Brewer's yeast, bran, organ meats, fish, chicken and meat	Aids in healing, growth and development
Vitamin B6	Brewers yeast, sunflower seeds, wheat germ, tuna liver, soybeans	Needed for blood component and protein production
Vitamin B12	Organ meats, clams, oysters, sardines, egg yolks, fish, cheese	Needed for blood cell production, bowel and nerve system health
Vitamin C	Peppers, kale, parsley, broccoli, brussels sprouts, citrus fruits and juices	For blood vessels, teeth and gums, antioxidant
Vitamin D	Sardines, salmon, tuna, shrimp, sunflower seeds, milk, eggs, cheese	Helps with calcium and phosphorus absorption
Vitamin E	Wheat germ, nuts, cooking oils, peanut butter, oatmeal	Antioxidant (has many beneficial properties)
Vitamin K	Green vegetables, cheese, liver, butter, milk, eggs	Assists in blood clotting

THE BOTTOM LINE

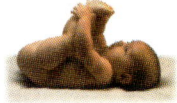

- Carpe diem! Seize the moment–with your children. Enjoy them while they last, for they don't stay children long enough.
- Prioritize your new life. Make yourself a top priority.
- Be kind and patient with yourself.
- Allow yourself time to grow into your new mother role.
- The true beauty of children is they forgive our mistakes, ignore our imperfections and love us without limits.
- Deal with difficulties as bumps before they become mountains.
- Learn to Drop, Delay and Delegate.
- Fatigue will be your nemesis for at least the first year.
- Learn to sleep when your baby sleeps.
- Ask for help. Accept help.
- Keep it simple. Don't complicate motherhood with minutia.
- Keep your partner "in the loop." Involve him in all parts of your new child's care.
- Encourage your partner to be an active participant, not a passive bystander. Give him time alone with baby so he can learn how to parent too.
- Parenting is a team sport. Don't make it an individual event.
- Keep the romance alive. Find time just for mom and dad.
- Love them and feed them. The rest will often handle itself.
- Learn to enjoy life again through your child's wonder and joy.
- Everyone has a different "mothering" style. You are unique, so develop your own style and flare. Make it special.
- Don't compare yourself to someone else. You'll only disappoint yourself.
- Learn to develop and trust your parents' intuition.
- Strive to become a medically aware and prepared mother.
- Above all else, believe in and trust yourself.
- Trying your best is all that matters in child rearing.
- Rely on your family doctor. Your family doctor should be your sounding board for all questions or concerns. Remember, there is no such thing as a stupid question!
- Keep your sense of humor. It will serve you well.
- Your life and body will be changed forever. Accept it.
- Breastfeed as long as you can. It really is the best choice.
- Have a great time and your children will too.

Parenting is a journey, not a guided tour.

FATHERHOOD (SURVIVAL STRATEGIES)

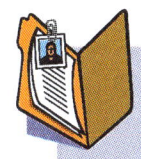

CASE STUDY

Mohammed came into the office with his wife at the two-week baby checkup of their first child.

After the baby's exam Mohammed lagged behind to discuss an important issue.

"I feel like I'm all thumbs," he admitted. "I haven't had much experience with babies and I don't know what to do. My wife on the other hand seems so much more comfortable than I am when looking after our child. I want to be an involved hands-on dad, but I just don't know what to do or when to do it. Do you think I am being illogical?"

I told Mohammed that good parents are developed, not delivered. I praised his initiative to become an active, involved father. I recommended a couple of books and Web sites. Most important, I encouraged him to roll up his sleeves and get busy with baby care. I told him that parenting was best learned by doing, especially when assisted by a supportive family, friends and wife.

Mohammed went on to have three other children and became an excellent father and a mentor to other fathers.

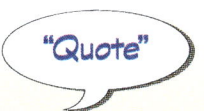

"Quote"

Fatherhood is like an Olympic training program.
"No pain, No gain."

You must become active and involved
to truly share in the joy of fatherhood.

Good fathers are made, not born.

FATHERHOOD (SURVIVAL STRATEGIES)

> **WARNING**
> *Talk to your Doctor/Mentor/Partner if you have ANY of the following:*
>
> - Feeling out of control, angry, depressed, scared, resentful, jealous, overwhelmed, left out or afraid of the baby.

SYMPTOMS

You may feel everything from euphoria to terror. The secret to fatherhood is to jump in and to get involved. Parenting is a team sport and you are an important part of the winning team.

FATHERHOOD TIPS (THE FIRST FEW WEEKS)

- Become active and involved from the very first day.
- Support your wife's recovery. Take time off or organize help (at least in the first few weeks after delivery).
- Your newborn may be quite different from what you imagined. Give baby and you time to get to know each other.
- Help with laundry, cooking, dishes, cleaning, groceries and other household chores. This is especially important when both partners work outside the home as well.
- Be supportive! Be patient! Be loving to your wife!
- Turn on the answering machine to screen calls. Tell people you will get back to them when things have "settled down."
- Limit the number of visitors and length of time they stay, especially in the first few weeks when mom and baby are trying to get to know each other's cues.
- Request all visitors bring food with them! Food is a great gift.
- Discuss important issues before they arise. Circumcision, bottle vs breastfeeding, how to deal with late-night feeds, illness during the day (and night), division of labor, etc.
- Be supportive of her breastfeeding. It is a learned, not innate, skill. Get her snacks and drinks, fetch the baby, change the diaper. Support from the husband is one of the most important factors in a woman continuing breastfeeding.
- Take a larger role in organizing the house and other children.
- Get home early to help out. Learn to balance work vs home.
- If in doubt, ask. There is no such thing as a stupid question when you are learning to be a great father.
- "Quality time" is a misnomer. Shoot for quantity and quality of time spent with your partner and children. To children, all time spent with their parents is considered quality time.
- Ask your partner what she would like you to do to help out. Despite what you may think, most mothers do not want to do it all themselves. Mothers love fathers to pitch in and help.
- Assist with the nighttime feedings.

FATHERHOOD (SURVIVAL STRATEGIES)

FATHERHOOD TIPS (THE FIRST FEW MONTHS)

- Keep the lines of communication open-talk about each other's feelings, anxieties, parenting styles and beliefs. Discuss differences in the way each of you were raised and what you would change in the way you were brought up.
- Make time for your relationship. (Remember, the one you had before she became pregnant.) Go on "dates" weekly. Learn to organize outings and babysitters. Keep the romance alive.
- Find a mentor (role model). Ask them what they did right and, more important, what they did wrong. Learn from their mistakes and the mistakes of others.
- Many new fathers have never had the opportunity of looking after a baby before. This makes becoming a father very scary. Have a friend or relative show you the basics with their baby before you take on your own-like diapering, bathing, etc.
- Expect your priorities to change… significantly.
- Just do your best. Parenting is like learning to walk. You always need a little extra time and practice.
- Fathers have unique stresses. Providing for the family, worries about becoming a father, worries about the health of mother and baby, fear of losing their relationship with their partner, jealousy of the mother getting all the attention and her infatuation with baby. These are all normal concerns. Talk openly to your mentor and partner about your concerns.
- Mothers can be too busy or too concerned about others to ask for help. Ask them what you can do to help out.
- Helping will give you a new challenge involving an individual that you helped create. It may be stressful at first, as learning any new skill is, but you will soon find that you excel at it.
- If your wife is driving you crazy with her overbearing management style, ask her calmly and politely to leave so you can practice on your own, with your baby, just like she did. (This is assuming you have already learned the skills needed.)
- Make time for you and baby to learn about each other.
- Help with nighttime feeds. If bottle feeding, either alternate feeds or nights so you both can get some sleep.
- Do special and unexpected things to keep the romance alive.
- Fathers can get postpartum depressions too. If you find yourself developing symptoms of depression (see page 57), get help.
- True parent – child "bonding" occurs not at birth but through the succeeding decades of caring for your child's needs.
- Feeling a little left out, jealous or inadequate? This is normal for many new fathers. Learn to perform a strong supporting role during this early performance. Your starring role will return.

YOUR HOME DOCTOR™ Mom　　167

FATHERHOOD (SURVIVAL STRATEGIES)

Trade Secrets

- Realize that your life is going to change. Recognize that this change will generally be for the better, not worse.
- Maintain contact with your friends and co-workers, even if this means a quick phone call once a month. Let them know you are still alive.
- Your relationship with your parents may change. Now you have one more thing to discuss and to make you closer.
- Your relationship with your wife will change. Expect this. Allow yourself time to slip into the new role of father.
- Being a good father means being a good provider. Remember to provide financially, emotionally, physically and spiritually.
- Being a mother is the most demanding job in the world. Regardless of your work requirements, your wife needs your help. Be an active participant not a passive bystander.
- Depending upon your wife's birth experience, returning to sexual intimacy may take anywhere from two weeks to twelve months.
- Men often take a little longer to settle in to their new "father" role than mothers do. Be patient and kind to yourself.
- New fathers can also develop the "baby blues."
- Responsibility and practicality are important qualities of a father but it is the irrational play and irresponsibility that your children will remember best. Learn to play. Be a kid again!
- The happenings of today will be gone tomorrow. Today's disaster is tomorrow's funny story at the water cooler.
- Read and learn at every opportunity. Educate yourself about kids.
- Caring and nurturing is not often a learned part of growing up male. Learn how to hold, diaper, soothe, bath and feed your baby.
Don't allow anyone to prevent you from experiencing the thrill of being a caring and nurturing father.
- Children are resilient. They love us despite our flaws.
- Be aware of your partner's needs.
- Be prepared to help out in any way possible.
- Be supportive. Be patient. Be loving. Have fun.
- Fathers should strive for three fundamental goals:
    - How to be a better father
    - How to be a better husband
    - How to be a better person

HOME FIRST AID/MEDICAL KIT

The Home First-Aid Kit

Every home should have a first-aid kit containing items appropriate for the ages of the family members. A first-aid kit in the home of a mother should contain at least the following.

Adhesive tape — For dressing wounds (use with gauze).
Bandage closures — In 5 mm (1/4 in.) and 2.5 cm (1 in.) sizes for taping edges of cuts together. (Also called "butterfly closures.")
Bandages — Assorted sizes for minor cuts and scrapes.
Child-safe ice pack — For injuries and treating fever.
First-Aid Manual — Should include a section on CPR
Gauze — In 5 and 10 cm (2 and 4 in.) widths for dressing wounds.
Gloves — Vinyl or latex for protecting hands and reducing the risk of infection when treating open wounds.
Heating pad or hot water bottle — Good for healing bruised soft tissues.
Peribottle — For spray cleansing the vagina and anus.
Safety pins — For fastening splints, slings and bandages.
Scissors — With rounded tips.
Triangular bandage — For wrapping bandages and making an arm sling.
Tweezers — For removing small splinters and ticks.

The Home First-Medical Kit

Acetaminophen — For pain, fever, and simple sprains and strains.
Antacids — For heartburn and indigestion.
Antibiotic cream — For burns, cuts and scrapes.
Antihistamines — For itching and allergies.
Anti-inflammatories — For pain, fever, muscle and ligament strains or sprains in non-breastfeeding moms.
Antinausea pills — For nausea and to help reduce vomiting.
Anti-yeast cream — To treat yeast infections.
Epsom salts — Add to bath for improved perineal and hemorrhoidal healing.
Fiber tabs — For constipation and hemorrhoids.
Hemorrhoid cream — To reduce hemorrhoid symptoms.
Saline nasal spray — For nasal congestion.
Skin moisturizer — For skin dryness and chapped hands.
Throat lozenges — For sore throats.
Vaporizer — For colds, nasal congestion and skin dryness. To increase a room's humidity.

Personal Information

Name: _____

Age: _____ Weight: _____

_____

Medication/Vitamins/Herbal Medicines: _____

_____

Allergies: _____

_____

Medical History: _____

_____

_____

_____

Surgical History: _____

_____

_____

Family History of Significance: _____

_____

Immunization Record (including last Tetanus shot): ___

_____

> The following two pages should be photocopied and completed for each individual in the family. A copy of these forms should be kept in a safe place. A copy of these forms should be brought to all medical appointments.

Record of Illness

Name: _____

Date: _____ Time: _____

Temperature: _____ Time: _____

Temperature: _____ Time: _____

Symptoms: _____

_____

_____

_____

_____

Home Treatment (list all medications used including herbal): _____

_____

_____

_____

_____

Diagnoses & Illness Duration: _____

_____

_____

Medical Treatment and Advice: _____

_____

_____

_____

_____

_____

Notes

Notes

Notes

Notes

Important Numbers

Emergency Services **911**

Hospital

Police

Fire

Ambulance

Poison Control

Family Doctor

Pharmacy

Breastfeeding Health Professional